Telemental Health in
Resource-Limited Global Settings

Telemental Health in Resource-Limited Global Settings

EDITED BY

HUSSAM JEFEE-BAHLOUL, MD
ASSISTANT PROFESSOR
UNIVERSITY OF MASSACHUSETTS MEDICAL SCHOOL
DEPARTMENT OF PSYCHIATRY
WORCESTER, MA

ANDRES BARKIL-OTEO, MD, MSC
CLINICAL ASSISTANT PROFESSOR OF PSYCHIATRY
YALE SCHOOL OF MEDICINE
NEW HAVEN, CT

EUGENE F. AUGUSTERFER, LCSW
DIRECTOR OF TELEMEDICINE
HARVARD PROGRAM IN REFUGEE TRAUMA
CAMBRIDGE, MA

OXFORD
UNIVERSITY PRESS

OXFORD
UNIVERSITY PRESS

Oxford University Press is a department of the University of Oxford. It furthers
the University's objective of excellence in research, scholarship, and education
by publishing worldwide. Oxford is a registered trade mark of Oxford University
Press in the UK and certain other countries.

Published in the United States of America by Oxford University Press
198 Madison Avenue, New York, NY 10016, United States of America.

CIP data is on file at the Library of Congress
ISBN 978–0–19–062272–5

9 8 7 6 5 4 3 2 1
Printed by Webcom, Inc., Canada

CONTENTS

CONTRIBUTORS   VII

1. Introduction to Telemental Health and Its Use
   in Resource-Limited Settings   1
   Hussam Jefee-Bahloul

2. Telemental Health Modalities: Videoconferencing, Store-and-Forward,
   Web-Based, and mHealth   15
   Jessica Becker

3. Telemental Health in Africa   33
   Sinclair Wynchank and Dora Wynchank

4. Telemental Health in South Africa   51
   Maurice Mars

5. Telemental Health in the Middle East   67
   Hussam Jefee-Bahloul and Zakaria Zayour

6. Telemental Health in India   89
   Rangaswamy Thara, Sujit John, and Kotteswara Rao

7. Telemental Health Services in Sri Lanka 105
   Sisira Edirippulige and Rohana B. Marasinghe

8. Telemental Health in Taiwan   117
   Hsiu-Hsin Tsai

9. Telemental Health Services for Indigenous Communities in Australia: A Work in Progress?   131
Sisira Edirippulige, Matthew Bambling, and Pablo Fernandez

10. Refugee Telemental Health in Denmark   145
Davor Mucic

11. Telemental Health Delivery for Rural Native American Populations in the United States   161
Shawn S. Sidhu, Chris Fore, Jay H. Shore, and Erin Tansey

12. Telemental Health in Latin America and the Caribbean   181
Tammi-Marie Phillip

13. Cross-Cultural Telemental Health   193
Niklas Skov Pape, Rasmus Christian Jørgensen, and Rune Weise Kofoed

14. Telemental Health in Postdisaster Settings   203
Eugene F. Augusterfer, Richard F. Mollica, and James Lavelle

15. Connecting the World: A Way Forward in Global Telemental Health   217
Juan Rodriguez Guzman and Andres Barkil-Oteo

INDEX   223

Eugene F. Augusterfer, LCSW
Director of Telemedicine
Harvard Program in
  Refugee Trauma
Cambridge, MA, USA

Matthew Bambling, PhD
PG Coursework Director
University of Queensland School
  of Medicine
Brisbane, Queensland, Australia

Andres Barkil-Oteo, MD, MSc
Clinical Assistant Professor of
  Psychiatry
Yale School of Medicine
New Haven, CT, USA

Jessica Becker, MD
Department of Psychiatry
Massachuessetts General Hospital
Harvard School of Medicine
Boston, MA, USA

Sisira Edirippulige, PhD, MPH
Senior Lecturer
Centre for Online Health
University of Queensland
Princess Alexandra Hospital
Brisbane, Australia

Pablo Fernandez, PhD Candidate
School of Psychology
University of Queensland
Australia

Chris Fore, PhD
Director, TeleBehavioral Health
  Center of Excellence
Division of Behavioral Health
Indian Health Service
Oklahoma State University
Albuquerque, NM, USA

Juan Rodriguez Guzman, MD
Department of Psychiatry
Yale University School of Medicine
New Haven, CT, USA

Hussam Jefee-Bahloul, MD
Assistant Professor
Department of Psychiatry
University of Massachussetts
  Medical School
Worcester, MA, USA

Sujit John, MA
Assistant Director
Schizophrenia Research
  Foundation (SCARF)
Chennai, India

Rasmus Christian Jørgensen
Graduate student in Psychology
  and Informatics
Roskilde University
Roskilde, Denmark

Rune Weise Kofoed
Graduate student in Game Design
IT University of Copenhagen
Copenhagen, Denmark

James Lavelle, LICSW
Co-Founder, Harvard Program in
  Refugee Trauma
Cambridge, MA, USA

Rohana B. Marasinghe, PhD
Senior Lecturer
University of Sri Jayewardenepura
Sri Lanka

Maurice Mars, MBChB, MD
Professor and Head of TeleHealth
College of Health Sciences
University of KwaZula-Natal
Durban, South Africa

Richard F. Mollica, MD, MAR
Professor of Psychiatry, Harvard
  Medical School
Director, Harvard Program in
  Refugee Trauma
Cambridge, MA, USA

Davor Mucic, MD
Little Prince Treatment Centre
Copenhagen, Denmark

Niklas Skov Pape, BS
Bachelor of Science in
  Communication and
  Informatics
Roskilde University
Roskilde, Denmark

Tammi-Marie Phillip, MD
Child Study Center
Yale School of Medicine
New Haven, CT, USA

Kotteswara Rao, MPhil
Senior Community Mental Health
  Coordinator
Schizophrenia Research
  Foundation (SCARF)
Chennai, India

Jay H. Shore, MD, MPH
Native Domain Lead
Veterans Rural Health
  Resource Center
Salt Lake City, UT, USA

Shawn S. Sidhu, MD
Associate Training Director,
  Rural and Community
  Training
UNM General Psychiatry
  Residency Program
Assistant Medical Director,
  UNM-IHS
Telebehavioral Health Center of
  Excellence Contract
Assistant Professor
University of New Mexico
  Department of Psychiatry
Albuquerque, NM, USA

Erin Tansey, MD
Attending Psychiatrist
Minneapolis, MN, USA

Rangaswamy Thara, MD, PhD,
  FRCPsych (Hon)
Director
Schizophrenia Research
  Foundation (SCARF)
Chennai, India

Hsiu-Hsin Tsai, RN, PhD
Associate Professor
School of Nursing, College of
  Medicine
Chang Gung University
Department of Psychiatry
Chang Gung Memorial Hospital
Tao-Yuan, Taiwan

Dora Wynchank, MBChB, MMed,
  FCPsych (SA)
PsyQ Expertise Center,
  Adult ADHD
The Hague, Netherlands

Sinclair Wynchank, MA, C Eng,
  MB, ChB, MD, DPhil
Strategic Health Innovation
  Partnerships
Medical Research Council of
  South Africa
Faculty of Health Sciences
University of Cape Town
Cape Town, South Africa

Zakaria Zayour, MD
Department of Psychiatry
University of Texas Southwestern
  Medical Center
Dallas, TX, USA

Introduction to Telemental Health and Its Use in Resource-Limited Settings

HUSSAM JEFEE-BAHLOUL

Let me tell you a story that comes from my imagination but is one that happens daily. Mr. R is a young man who lives with his family in Pudukottai, a rural district in southern India. He is the only child of an elderly father and mother. Both parents have health concerns and poor mobility. Mr. R started to withdraw socially few years back and had episodes of anger, during one of which he once assaulted a neighbor. He was taken to a religious healer in the town with no effect. He started to hear voices and told his mother secretly that he thinks his neighbors are conspiring against him. He had times during which he would refuse to eat for days despite the family's relentless efforts to make him eat. He also had periods where he did not sleep and stayed up all night. His parents wanted to find a solution. The closest psychiatrist is more than 150 kilometers away, and travel for the family is almost impossible. Besides the lack of financial means, the parents are also too weak to tolerate such a long trip.

For someone like Mr. R, the options are limited. His family could wait until travel is more feasible, but this risks deterioration of his mental state and worsening of his dangerous behavior. He could try to see a medical doctor in the area, but chances are the medical provider will have limited knowledge and training to make a diagnosis, maintain rapport with this vulnerable patient, and execute an effective treatment plan.

One day, R's cousin came home to talk about what he had heard. "A bus that has a screen . . . a psychiatrist is seen through the screen . . . a doctor who is kilometers away!" the cousin said. It felt like the perfect match for Mr. R. The bus travels and visits his town periodically.

In 2005, a program called Schizophrenia Research Foundation (SCARF) found a way to provide mental healthcare to severely ill patients in India. SCARF's mobile telepsychiatry service is provided on a bus that was custom built to contain a consultation room and a pharmacy. In the consultation room, communication takes place between the patients and psychiatrists based in the city of Chennai, more than 450 km away. After a teleconsultation, and with a diagnosis being reached, a prescription is dictated by the psychiatrist to the telepsychiatry clinic facilitator in the bus and is fulfilled by the on-board pharmacy. A follow-up appointment date is given, at which medication is reviewed and further treatment provided.

Mr. R visited the bus, had an evaluation with a psychiatrist via video-conferencing, and left with a prescription of an antipsychotic, as there was no indication of dangerousness. He received the medications for free from the same bus. The next week, a community lay worker affiliated with SCARF made a home visit to make sure Mr. R was taking medications as prescribed and had no major concerns. Weeks later Mr. R started to be more active around the house and became more social with his cousins. In the case of Mr. R, like thousands of other cases, technology improved the odds of his accessing quality of mental healthcare. According to Dr. Thara of SCARF, "There are only 4,000 psychiatrists in India, 70 per cent of whom are in urban areas, leaving the vast majority without access to mental health facilities. Telemedicine offers a unique way to fill this gap in services."[1]

Let us take another example—Ahmad, a healthcare provider in a remote clinic near the Syrian Turkish borders. Ahmad has a bachelor's degree in psychology from Syria, but had no clinical experience providing mental healthcare before the war. After the war started, he was forced to flee his home to a new city where he was recruited by a humanitarian organization to help see patients who presented to a primary care clinic and happened to ask to see a mental healthcare provider. He was recruited because there were no psychiatrists or other mental healthcare providers available in that remote area. Syria lacked a mental health infrastructure before the war. The war only made things worse. One day, Ahmad was in the clinic when a mother came in with her 6-year-old boy complaining that the boy would not sit still all day. The mother noted that her child's verbal abilities were deteriorating, and he was not able to say and repeat things he used to say in the past, such as many verses of the Quran that he had memorized when he was 4 years old. The mother states that all of these issues started a year ago when they were still in Aleppo and there was a lot of bombing and active fighting. His developmental history was normal until the onset of his current condition. He was seen in a healthcare center elsewhere and they diagnosed him with autism. He was prescribed risperidone, but the family never gave it to him.

Ahmad examined the child, tried to talk to him, but noticed that the child's verbal abilities were not as expected at his age and he was also hyperactive. Ahmad was not sure of the diagnosis. Could it be autism? Maybe, he thought, but he remembered reading that autistic children do not maintain good eye contact with people. This child was responding physically to people around him. Could it be something else? He had no clue. His training and background were lacking when it came to such complex cases. There was no child psychiatrist is this area. The closest might be in Turkey. And good luck finding an Arabic-speaking child psychiatrist in Turkey, he thought to himself.

With the mother's permission, he took a short video clip of the child using his smart phone. The clip consisted of the mother trying to communicate with her child and the child's reactions to his mother. He asked the mother to come back with the child next week. Later that day, he uploaded the videos and wrote up the clinical case on Collegium Telemedicus. This is the platform that connects Ahmad and dozens of healthcare providers like him in the Syrian humanitarian scene with mental health specialists around the world using telemedicine. This is a different form of telemedicine compared with our earlier story from India. This "store-and-forward" system allows Ahmad and providers like him to provide clinical materials and transmit them through a secure platform to get specialized advice, otherwise unavailable. Less than 24 hours later, he received an e-mail indicating that a response to his case was awaiting him on the platform. The case has been allocated to a Syrian child and adolescent psychiatrist who was trained and practicing in the United States. Based on the clinical material provided, the onset after trauma, the child's behavior in the video, and his social interactions (especially his ability to communicate verbally to with his mother and maintain eye contact), all indicated a traumatic reaction rather than an autistic disorder. A treatment plan was set in motion, to focus on family education, supportive psychotherapy, involvement of the whole family in his care, and possibly low doses of antidepressant and melatonin to help him sleep. The consultant also provided educational material for Ahmad to read about complex reactions to traumas in children. Weeks after the first visitation the child started to improve, and the family was happier with the progress. Most importantly, Ahmad, as a provider, now felt more confident of his diagnosis and treatment plan, was more educated about this child's case, and had an ongoing channel of communication with an expert in this child's case. All thanks to technology.

At the heart of global health lies the most burdensome and "heavy weight" challenger: global mental health. Contrary to common perception, mental health causes more global suffering than cardiovascular disease or cancer.[2] Mental and substance use disorders account for 7.4% of the world's burden of health conditions in terms of disability-adjusted life-years.[3]

In the field of mental health, there is an enormous gap between knowledge and delivery of evidence-based healthcare. According to the World Health Organization (WHO) mental health Gap Action Program (mhGAP), there is robust evidence for the effectiveness of a biopsychosocial interventions in the field of mental health—these interventions "can transform lives and enhance communities."[2,4] While this is true, the majority of the world's population has no access to these interventions (see Table 1.1 for information regarding mental health services globally based on a *Lancet* report by Jacob et al.[5]). Innovative strategies that overcome the barriers to provision of mental healthcare are essential to increase access and improve the lives of millions affected by mental illness.[6] The use of technology has been identified as one of the innovations capable of bridging this provisional gap. According to Patel et al., "Technology can play a key part ... for example, by enhancing access to specialist care by means of telemedicine, enhancing adherence and follow-up with the use of mobile phones, and creating opportunities for self-care by means of Internet-delivered treatment."[2]

Telemental health (TMH) is a broad concept that defines delivery of mental health services using technological means. While TMH includes a lot of synonyms such as "telepsychiatry," "telepsychology," "e-mental health," "mobile health," and others, all the terms focus on one idea: the delivery of mental health services at a distance.[7] These services include clinical care, consultation, education, training, or research. In other words, TMH can provide services including diagnosis and treatment of patients; education of staff, patients, and the general public; administrative activities, such as collecting public health data; and research.

Telemental health can help increase access in many ways, including reducing the need to travel, especially in areas where mental health services are concentrated in large urban settings, so patients in remote areas face the burden of traveling to receive quality care. As we saw in the first story in this chapter, the SCARF project in India is an example of how telemedicine (and in this sense TMH) via videoconferencing can help increase access for mentally ill patients who otherwise have no access to mental health services. Also, TMH can increase the speed by which a specialist's opinion can be obtained, as we saw in the second story, which was an example of our work at the Syrian Telemental Health Network (STMH). In the STMH a consultative network using "store-and-forward" technology (discussed in detail in chapter 2) was used to provide tertiary consultation for humanitarian field healthcare workers in the Syrian crisis. At times, healthcare workers needed specialized opinions

TABLE 1.1 MENTAL HEALTH SERVICES CHARACTERISTICS OF SAMPLE
COUNTRIES FROM DIFFERENT WORLD REGIONS

	Proportion of mental health budget (% of total health budget)	Suicide per 100,000 people	Total numbers of mental health beds per 10,000	Number of psychia-trists per 100,000	Number of psychiatric nurses per 100,000
AFRICA					
Algeria	..	2.87	1.4	1.1	1.1
Cameroon	0.1	4.75	0.08	0.03	0.2
Dem. Rep. of the Congo	..	4.79	0.17	0.04	0.03
Rep. of the Congo	..	6.31	0.06	0.03	0.1
Ethiopia	..	3.49	0.07	0.02	0.3
Ghana	0.5	3.95	1.03	0.08	2
Kenya	0.01	5.94	0.4	0.2	2
Madagascar	0.82	4.28	0.17	0.08	0.3
Nigeria	..	4.93	0.4	0.09	4
South Africa	..	10.55	4.5	1.2	7.5
Uganda	0.7	2.01	0.44	1.6	2
Zambia	..	3.36	0.5	0.02	5
AMERICA					
Argentina	..	10.21	6	13.25	..
Brazil	2.5	5	2.56	4.8	..
Canada	..	11.75	19.3	12	44
Australia	9.6	11.31	3.9	14	53
Honduras	2.3	8.1	0.6	0.76	0
Panama	..	5	2.55	3.7	5
USA	6	10.34	7.7	13.7	6.5

TABLE 1.1 CONTINUED

	Proportion of mental health budget (% of total health budget)	Suicide per 100,000 people	Total numbers of mental health beds per 10,000	Number of psychiatrists per 100,000	Number of psychiatric nurses per 100,000
EUROPE					
Denmark		13.36	7.1	16	59
Finland		23.38	10	22	180
France		15.92	12	22	98
Germany		13.88	7.5	11.8	52
Italy		6.78	4.6	9.8	32.9
Netherlands		8.89	18.7	9	99
Norway		11.34	12	20	42
Russia		40.96	11.5	13.3	50
Sweden		12.8	6	20	32
Switzerland		17.9	13.2	23	46
UK		8.45	5.8	11	104
MIDDLE EAST					
Bahrain	..	4.37	3.3	5	23
Cyprus	7	16.25	13.46	5	45
Egypt	9	1.51	1.3	0.9	2
Iran	3	8.22	1.6	1.9	0.5
Iraq	..	6.88	0.6	0.7	0.1
Israel	6.2	4.78	8.1	13.7	10.7
Jordan	..	17.17	1.5	1	2
Kuwait	..	1.78	3.4	3.1	22.5
Lebanon	..	6.05	7.5	2	5.3
Oman	..	4.04	0.4	1.4	5
Qatar	1	4.47	0.9	3.4	10

(continued)

TABLE 1.1 CONTINUED

	Proportion of mental health budget (% of total health budget)	Suicide per 100,000 people	Total numbers of mental health beds per 10,000	Number of psychia-trists per 100,000	Number of psychiatric nurses per 100,000
Saudi Arabia	..	5.81	1.18	1.1	6.4
Syria	..	0.56	0.8	0.5	0.5
Tunisia	..	4.42	1.1	1.6	0.2
Turkey	..	6.67	1.3	1	3
UAE	..	3.81	1.4	2	11
Yemen	..	4.90	1.85	0.5	0.09
WEST PACIFIC					
Australia	9.6	11.31	3.9	14	53
China	2.35	20.94	1.06	1.29	1.99
New Zealand	11	12.2	3.8	6.6	74
South Korea	3	18.17	13.8	3.5	10.1
Vietnam	..	11.03	0.63	0.32	0.3
SOUTHEAST ASIA					
India	2.05	17.38	0.25	0.2	0.05
Indonesia	1	11.31	0.4	0.21	0.9

SOURCE: Numbers adapted from Jacob et al. (2007)[5]

on their difficult mental health cases, but they practiced in areas where no specialists were available for consultation. The telemental health network using a basic Internet connection made it possible for these workers to document cases they chose and transmit them to a psychiatrist located thousands of miles away, who would provide their opinion.

Cost-effectiveness for TMH in resource-limited settings lacks robust research, as no large-scale studies have been conducted or replicated so far. It is to be expected that findings would differ in each setting and context. For example in chapter 6, we see that a cost-effectiveness analysis of a videoconferencing-based TMH program in Israel was found to be more expensive than regular care. More cost-effective analysis studies are encouraged in each setting after the pilot phase and before scaling up programs.

Telemental health has two main modalities: real-time, live interaction (synchronous) and store-and-forward (asynchronous) technologies. Mobile health can be considered "synchronous" when direct communication with providers is facilitated by the mobile phones, or "asynchronous" if beneficiaries are receiving data that has been recorded and then sent (via text messages or smart phone apps) (Table 1.2). Chapters 2 and 3 provide a general overview of telemedicine and TMH, including a description of modalities and their applicability in providing clinical and educational services. It is worth noting that while videoconferencing-based TMH is possible in resource-limited environments, it is also the case that nonsynchronous (store-and-forward) telemedicine is more common in these settings, not only because it is usually cheaper but also because the nonsynchronous nature of the interaction among the parties makes it easier to organize. Chapters in this book highlight both modalities.

Finally, the term "resource-limited settings" covers most low-income countries and also includes regions in middle- or high-income countries where underserved populations have difficulties in accessing specialists.[7] In this book, we present a selection of chapters that showcase TMH programs in some of these resource-limited settings. There exists a wider range of reports from different regions in the world, and it is beyond the scope of this book to provide a comprehensive review of those reports. Rather, the major aim of this book is to provide examples of global implementation of TMH in resource-limited settings. This demonstration will allow mental health providers, researchers, policymakers, and anyone who is invested in relieving the global burden of mental illness to consider the role of technology in bridging the existing provisional gap.

The following chapters provide examples of the global applicability of TMH modalities in different resource-limited settings. Chapters present reports from low- and middle-income countries such as India, Sri Lanka,

TABLE 1.2 GLOBAL EXAMPLES OF TELEMENTAL HEALTH MODALITIES FOR DIFFERENT UTILITIES

	Patient care	Consultations	Training	Education	Research
Live interaction (synchronous TMH)	India: SCARF project[8] Somaliland: Expatriate TMH project[9] South Africa: Nursing support project[10] South Africa: (KwaZulu-Natal) Multidistrict VC TMH project[11] Taiwan: Tsai, VC nursing homes[12] Israel: Or Akiva study[13] Sri Lanka: CCCline phone counseling.[14]	South Africa: Regional Hospital outreach project[15]	Kenya: African MH Foundation training to Somali providers.[16] Jordan: telesupervision in humanitarian setting.[17]	Africa: Pan-African eNetwork South Africa: teaching psychiatry registrars by VC.[18] Turkey: psycho-education for family members by phone.[19]	

Store-and-forward (asynchronous TMH)			
(4) South Africa: Antenatal depression project[20]	(5) Syria: STMH Network. S&F teleconsultative system in Syria.[25]	(4) South Africa: University of KwaZulu-Natal videorecorded outreach lectures[15]	(4) South Africa: Project "Masihambisane"[27] using mobile in collecting research data.
(4) South Africa: Cellphones4Africa in HIV + women[21]		(7) Sri Lanka: "Health Net" program, public education on mental health.[26]	
(8) Taiwan: Cybercounseling reports[22]			
(5) Iraq: Interpay CBT[23]			
(7) Sri Lanka: "Sahana" project.[24]			

Numbers indicate the chapter numbers in which these examples can be found.

NOTE: Projects listed here are only demonstrative examples to the broad spectrum of TMH and its global applicability. This list of projects is not inclusive of all reported experiences.

Taiwan, the Middle East, Africa, and Latin America. Other chapters report from high-income countries, focusing on outreach programs to under-served populations. Chapter 10 describes TMH services for indigenous people in Australia, chapter 11 describes TMH for refugees in Sweden and Denmark, and chapter 12 describes existing experience in providing TMH services for Native American populations in the United States.

REFERENCES

1. Mobile rural tele-psychiatry initiative launched. 2011. http://www.thehindu. com/news/cities/chennai/mobile-rural-telepsychiatry-initiative-launched/article1200593.ece. Accessed July 15, 2015.
2. Patel V, Saxena S. Transforming lives, enhancing communities: innovations in global mental health. New England Journal of Medicine. 2014;370(6):498–501.
3. Whiteford HA, Degenhardt L, Rehm J, et al. Global burden of disease attributable to mental and substance use disorders: findings from the Global Burden of Disease Study 2010. Lancet. 2013;382(9904):1575–1586.
4. World Health Organization. Mental Health Gap Action Programme: MhGAP intervention guide for mental, neurological and substance use disorders in non-specialized health settings: Version 1.0. World Health Organization. 2010.
5. Jacob K, Sharan P, Mirza I, et al. Mental health systems in countries: where are we now? Lancet. 2007;370(9592):1061–1077.
6. Rebello TJ, Marques A, Gureje O, Pike KM. Innovative strategies for closing the mental health treatment gap globally. Current Opinion in Psychiatry. 2014;27(4):308–314.
7. Wootton R, Bonnardot L. Telemedicine in low-resource settings. Frontiers in Public Health. 2015;3:3.
8. Thara R, John S, Rao K. Telepsychiatry in Chennai, India: the SCARF experience. Behavioral Sciences and the Law. 2008;26(3):315–322.
9. Abdi YA, Elmi JY. Internet based telepsychiatry: a pilot case in Somaliland. Medicine, Conflict and Survival. 2011;27(3):145–150.
10. Wynchank S, Fortuin J. Telenursing in Africa. In: Kumar S Snooks H, ed. Telenursing. 1st ed. London: Springer; 2011:119–129.
11. Chipps J, Ramlall S, Madigoe T, King H, Mars M. Developing telepsychiatry services in KwaZulu-Natal: an action research study. African Journal of Psychiatry. 2012;15(4):255–263.
12. Tsai H-H, Tsai Y-F, Wang H-H, Chang Y-C, Chu HH. Videoconference program enhances social support, loneliness, and depressive status of elderly nursing home residents. Aging and Mental Health. 2010;14(8):947–954.

13. Modai I, Jabarin M, Kurs R, Barak P, Hanan I, Kitain L. Cost effectiveness, safety, and satisfaction with video telepsychiatry versus face-to-face care in ambulatory settings. Telemedicine Journal and e-Health. 2006;12(5):515–520.

14. CCC Foundation. CCCline. http://cccfoundation.org.au/cccline/. Accessed July 26, 2015.

15. Chipps J, Ramlall S, Mars M. A telepsychiatry model to support psychiatric outreach in the public sector in South Africa. African Journal of Psychiatry. 2012;15(4):264–270.

16. Ndetei D. Tele-Psychiatry between Nairobi and Somalia 2010. https://www.rcpsych.ac.uk/docs/Newsletter%20March%202010%20(2).doc.

17. Jefee-Bahloul H. Use of telepsychiatry in areas of conflict: the Syrian refugee crisis as an example. Journal of Telemedicine and Telecare. 2014;20(3):165–166.

18. Chipps J, Ramlall S, Mars M. Videoconference-based education for psychiatry registrars at the University of KwaZulu-Natal, South Africa. African Journal of Psychiatry. 2012;15(4).

19. Ozkan B, Erdem E, Ozsoy SD, Zararsiz G. Effect of psychoeducation and telepsychiatric follow up given to the caregiver of the schizophrenic patient on family burden, depression and expression of emotion. Pakistan Journal of Medical Sciences. 2013;29(5):1122.

20. Tsai AC, Tomlinson M, Dewing S, et al. Antenatal depression case finding by community health workers in South Africa: feasibility of a mobile phone application. Archives of Women's Mental Health. 2014;17(5):423–431.

21. Déglise C, Suggs LS, Odermatt P. Short message service (SMS) applications for disease prevention in developing countries. Journal of Medical Internet Research. 2012;14(1):e3.

22. Li W-P, Chen C-F, Wang C-H. Agreements on working alliance and session impact in cybercounseling and interview counseling. Bulletin of Educational Psychology. 2008.

23. Wagner B, Schulz W, Knaevelsrud C. Efficacy of an Internet-based intervention for posttraumatic stress disorder in Iraq: a pilot study. Psychiatry Research. 2012;195(1–2):85–88.

24. Careem M, De Silva C, De Silva R, Raschid L, Weerawarana S. Sahana: overview of a disaster management system. Paper presented at Information and Automation International Conference on Dec. 15–17, 2006.

25. Syrian Telemental Health Network (STMH). 2015. www.stmh.net. Accessed July 13, 2015.

26. Suwasariya (Health Net). Health Education Bureau Ministry of Health—Sri Lanka. http://suwasariya.gov.lk/index.php?option=com_info&id=7&task=cat&Itemid=11&lang=en. Accessed July 26, 2015.

27. Rotheram-Borus MJ, Tomlinson M, le Roux IM, et al. A cluster randomised controlled effectiveness trial evaluating perinatal home visiting among South African mothers/infants. PLoS ONE. 2014;9(10):e105934.

2

Telemental Health Modalities

*Videoconferencing, Store-and-Forward,
Web-Based, and mHealth*

JESSICA BECKER

Telemental health (TMH) around the globe has grown to rely on the use of videoconferencing technology. Whereas telemedicine more generally can often rely on voice and static images, such as a dermatologic consult on a skin lesion, TMH is particularly well suited to the dynamic visual and voice capabilities of video conferencing. Real-time visualization allows for provider analysis of a patient's verbal, physical, and nonverbal cues.[1,2]

Videoconferencing-based telemental health (VC-TMH) encrypted use of video conferencing technology to deliver mental healthcare at a distance. While traditionally videoconferencing was used primarily for consultation when a psychiatrist was not readily available,[3] its purposes have expanded to include psychiatric diagnosis, assessment, treatment, and maintenance.[1,3,4] In addition to acute diagnosis and management, VC-TMH has been used for longer-term psychotherapy sessions, particularly with cognitive-behavioral therapy (CBT).[5,6] Further, VC-TMH has been used beyond direct patient–provider interaction for remote psychiatric consultation to guide primary care physicians in diagnosis and treatment management in regions underserved by mental health specialists.[5,6] Telemental health, and particularly VC-TMH, is an important venue for widening the reach of mental health professionals to alleviate shortages of specialty care in a cost-effective way.[6,7]

This chapter begins with a discussion of the technical basics of VC-TMH setup and a brief consideration of other technologies in TMH such as store-and-forward and mobile health. It addresses the effectiveness of VC-TMH in the United States and internationally, including a discussion of recent data evaluating VC-TMH use. The chapter concludes with a discussion of the challenges facing implementation of TMH in the United States and abroad, including policy, technical, infrastructure, financial, and patient-safety concerns.

VIDEOCONFERENCING-BASED TELEMENTAL HEALTH

This section details the technology needed for optimal VC-TMH connection and quality.

Basic Set-up

The standard setup for a VC-TMH system allows for ample audiovisual interaction between the patient and provider. The video system therefore should consist of the use of a video camera, microphone, speakers, headset, and viewing monitors on both the patient and provider side.[1] A camera with pan, tilt, and zoom features is particularly useful for allowing an optimal view of patient and provider,[6,7] though even a simple webcam can be used.[1] Note that the video camera can be provided via personal computer or mobile device, such as a "smartphone."[7] The advent of the laptop and tablet allows for additional flexibility for patients and providers.

Network Connection

Early models of VC-TMH systems used closed-circuit televisions or secure, point-to-point network connections over telephone lines, known as T1 or Integrated Services Digital Network (ISDN) circuits.[1,8] More modern VC-TMH systems, however, generally use Internet protocol (IP) networks. Unlike the earlier T1 and ISDN circuits, IP networks are not secure and therefore require the use of encryption, a virtual private network (VPN) setup, or a virtual local area network (VLAN) setup in order to protect patient privacy.[1] On the other hand, IP networks have the advantage of being usable by multiple applications at once and can therefore connect patient and provider systems over Internet, e-mail, local area networks (LANs), and other applications simultaneously.[1] In order to maintain a reliable Internet connection for an IP network, wired Internet is preferable to wireless when available.[7]

Audio Quality

Given the importance of dialogue in a psychiatric assessment and treatment encounter, high-quality audio is imperative in VC-TMH, particularly during direct patient–provider remote interactions. Audio transmission can be improved through the use of high-quality microphones and speakers.[6] It is also important to consider the placement of the microphones and speakers at either end of the line, as well as the room acoustics for both patient and provider to ensure optimal communication.[6]

Video Quality

Video quality, measured in frames per second, indicates how closely the VC-TMH video will match to real time. Lower-quality video has fewer frames per second and can lead to a "flickering image."[1] This in turn can lead to difficulty visualizing movements and expression from both the patient and provider perspective,[1] which can affect the provider's evaluation of the patient's state and can pose consequences to both parties' interpretation of affect during a TMH encounter. In the context of international VC-TMH, cross-cultural TMH encounters may pose additional challenges with the possibility of different cultural interpretations of eye contact and body language between the patient and provider's home cultures.[9] Given these considerations, the suggested minimum speed for VC-TMH sessions is 30 frames per second.[7] Additionally, videoconferencing software continues to be improved to bolster signal quality over IP networks; such protocols are usually embedded in the actual videoconferencing systems and can improve the quality of VC-TMH encounter transmission.[6]

Given the particularly high importance of interpersonal interaction in psychiatric care, VC-TMH systems have generally relied on high-bandwidth networks.[1] Bandwidth indicates the amount of data that can be transmitted or received over a network, with a higher transmission rate leading to a shorter delay in audiovisual signal.[1] There has been some evidence to show that increasing videoconferencing bandwidth, and therefore improving the audiovisual quality of VC-TMH, may lead to increased uptake of VC-TMH and reduction in psychiatric emergency room visits.[10,11] Videoconferencing guidelines suggest Internet-based videoconferencing software that runs at a bandwidth of 384 kilobits per second (Kbps) or higher in both downlink and uplink directions.[6,7] A bandwidth test can be used to test a connection before initiating a patient session to verify connection quality.[7]

Additionally, high bandwidth requires the need for a coder/decoder system, or codec, to conserve bandwidth during transmission.[1,6] A codec converts analog audiovisual signal to digital audiovisual code, compresses the digital code for transmission, and decodes it for playback on the receiving end.[1,6] However, while codecs were previously an additional technological device, they are now generally standardly integrated into personal computers.[1]

Finally, once the audiovisual signal is received, the monitors used for display of a VC-TMH session should have a resolution that matches as closely as possible to the resolution of the transmitted image, in order to maximize picture quality.[6] The suggested minimum resolution for VC-TMH sessions is 640x360.[7] Further, as with audio considerations, room lighting and video placement within rooms are important to consider when devising maximal video quality in a VC-TMH encounter.[6]

Access to Patient Medical Record

In order to have full patient information for optimal VC-TMH consultation, the mental health provider will usually need access to additional patient information beyond the video data, such as access to the patient's record, transmission of an electronic medical record, or additional faxed or e-mailed patient data.[6] All such transmission of additional patient data must occur within the bounds of legal and regulatory requirements and privacy protections.[6]

EVIDENCE FOR TELEMENTAL HEALTH

This section summarizes the evidence that has taken shape for TMH thus far, with an emphasis on evidence for VC-TMH.

Evaluation

While the evidence base for VC-TMH is still growing, thus far it has generally been found to be comparable to in-person mental healthcare with regard to psychiatric assessment and treatment, as well as when considering structural issues such as feasibility and patient and provider satisfaction.[12] Further, there have been no studies to date that show either no benefit or particular harm to any subpopulation of patients undergoing VC-TMH, which underscores its likely generalizability.[7]

A 2005 comprehensive review of the literature between 1956 and 2002 found that only 14 studies with a cohort size over 10 participants had directly compared TMH to in-person mental healthcare, summing to 500 patients included in the meta-analysis.[11] The meta-analysis found no difference in objective assessment or satisfaction measures between in-person mental health encounters and TMH encounters.[11] Still, while promising, the sample size was relatively small, even combined.

More recent studies evaluating the implementation of TMH services in the United States have shown significant improvement in mental health outcomes with TMH.[5] The first large-scale study to examine TMH outcomes, a recent 4-year study of over 98,000 patients enrolled in high-speed VC-TMH services provided by the US Department of Veterans Affairs (VA), found a 24% decrease in psychiatric hospitalization rates and a 26% decrease in total hospitalization days after enrollment in VC-TMH services.[13] Though there was no direct comparison group in this study, the overall rate of psychiatric hospitalization of VA mental health patients increased during the time of the study, supporting the suggestion that the TMH intervention may explain the study's findings.[13]

Another 2007 study based in California demonstrated that converting a small telepsychiatric consultation service into a "virtual mental health clinic" by increasing capacity, adding e-mail and telephone consultations to previously existing video-based formats, adding a clinical psychologist to the consulting team, and adding in educational programming for primary care providers in rural settings led to significant improvements in the Mental Component Summary of the SF-12.[5] This study displays the broad capability of TMH interventions and their resulting efficacy.

Finally, a 2010 systematic review identified 10 randomized, controlled trials evaluating the use of videoconference as compared to in-person encounters for psychiatric diagnosis and treatment.[14] Of the seven reviewed studies evaluating outcomes, comprising 969 patients in total, symptoms were not significantly different between the intervention and control groups. In sum, this study, along with the others like it, supports the feasibility of, efficacy of, and patient satisfaction with VC-TMH.

Still, there remains work to be done in assessing outcomes of VC-TMH implementation; toward this end, a lexicon has been proposed to standardize evaluation of VC-TMH services.[15]

Specific Consideration of Psychiatric Illness

One important consideration for VC-TMH, as compared with telemedicine in general, is the possibility of exacerbating symptoms in patients who may perceive videoconferencing itself as challenging, such as those with psychotic or phobic disorders. One recent study suggests that VC-TMH is not inferior to in-person mental healthcare for patients with psychotic disorders,[7,8] while another demonstrates that even psychotic patients with delusions regarding television responded appropriately to VC-TMH and did not incorporate the sessions into their delusions.[7] Still, it is important when implementing or using TMH interventions to consider their effect on each individual patient.

OTHER TELEMENTAL HEALTH TECHNOLOGIES

While VC-TMH has been the core of TMH thus far, other TMH technologies have also been used with success. This section describes some of these other technologies and briefly discusses evidence in their evaluation.

Asynchronous Telemental Health

Asynchronous TMH allows the patient and provider to connect via telecommunications without talking or videoconferencing in real time.[2,16] Examples of this include communication over e-mail and store-and-forward strategies, which are described in detail here.

STORE-AND-FORWARD TECHNOLOGY
In a store-and-forward model, patient assessments in an underresourced area can be recorded on video and uploaded electronically via e-mail or a Web-based application for review by a psychiatrist remotely.[16] A store-and-forward telemedicine model was first studied in a TMH setting in 2010.[16] In this study, a cohort of 60 patients in medically underserved

areas in California were assessed by a local nonpsychiatrist physician on video in a nonemergent setting; the local physician then uploaded the video data and additional health data to a privacy-protected, Internet-based consultation electronic medical record.[16] The remote psychiatrist then reviewed the patient video and health data over the Web-based electronic medical record and provided formal consultant recommendations to the local physician, with availability to discuss the case over telephone or e-mail and to have the psychiatrist meet in person with the patient, if recommended by the consulting psychiatrist.[16] In this study, the remote psychiatrists recommended a short-term medication change to the local physician in 95% of the referred cases, along with a long-term suggested treatment plan with both medication and therapy suggestions.[16] These findings show the overwhelming impact that asynchronous TMH can have in improving patient care.

The same group went on to examine cross-language asynchronous telepsychiatric consultation, demonstrating the usefulness of videorecording over real-time or in-person consultation in improving access to proper translation, and showing moderate to very good agreement in assessment between same-language and other-language consultants with augmented translation.[17] While this initial evidence is promising for the use of asynchronous telepsychiatry in the international setting when translation is required between patient and provider, further work must be undertaken to understand how to control for cultural and linguistic differences in expressing psychiatric states when using cross-language TMH.[12]

Cost-Effectiveness

Data have been mixed on the costs and cost-effectiveness of synchronous, or real-time, telepsychiatry consultation, as compared with face-to-face patient encounters; theoretically, the same amount of time is spent with a patient in synchronous telepsychiatry as in a face-to-face encounter, but the additional costs of a high-quality, privacy-protected videoconferencing software and the availability of an adequate, secure Internet connection may make this method less cost-effective, depending on distance between patient and provider.[18] Asynchronous telepsychiatry, on the other hand, can replace the in-person specialist time with that of a medical assistant or other lower-cost health provider during the recorded patient assessment, which can bring down overall costs of this version of telepsychiatry.[18] Indeed, early data on costs of asynchronous telepsychiatry suggests that it is more cost-effective than in-person consultation or real-time TMH once 250 or more consultations are obtained.[18]

Mobile Technology

The onslaught of mobile telephone technology in recent years has also led to a new, and fast-growing, venue for TMH—the mobile phone. Telemental health practiced over mobile phones may be particularly important for regions of the world such as rural sub-Saharan Africa, where a stable power supply and Internet access may be less accessible than mobile phones.[19] Uses for mobile phones include both synchronous communication between patient and provider and asynchronous methods of TMH, such as through text message or mobile phone applications ("apps").

In recent years, thousands of mobile telephone "apps" have been created to fill the void of access to mental healthcare.[4] Apps have been created to complement many stages along the care pathway, from diagnostic assistance to maintenance with self-monitoring and symptom tracking to reminders for medication, appointments, and therapy homework to improve patient adherence to treatment.[4] Mobile therapy apps have been also been created to encourage self-awareness and to administer CBT-like therapy.[4]

While not yet well studied, preliminary evidence from several small randomized, controlled trials suggests clinical improvements among patients using self-monitoring and CBT-based apps.[4] Still, among the thousands of apps in existence, a recent review found that only eight were evidence-based, and of these, only two were available for public download.[20] Thus, there are still needs for guidelines and quality control measures before app-based TMH becomes more widespread. Additionally, while apps are promising in their portability and usefulness in tracking behavioral data over time, their limitations in terms of attrition and respondent fatigue must be better evaluated to inform their true efficacy.[4]

As discussed, another form of mobile TMH, while not yet rigorously studied, is text messaging, or short message service (SMS). As with apps, SMS can be used synchronously or asynchronously as a way for clinicians to connect with patients, as well as to send reminders of goals, appointments, and therapy homework.[4]

Internet-based Interventions

Asynchronous TMH can also take place through Internet-based interventions. Among the best described such methods is Internet-based cognitive-behavioral therapy (iCBT).

Due to its generally standardized nature, CBT has been thought of as a form of therapy well suited to delivery systems with minimal therapist involvement, such as over the Internet or mobile phones.[4] From the 1980s, computer software has been used to administer automated CBT directly to patients.[4] With the advent of the Internet age, tele-CBT can take the form of asynchronous Internet-based unassisted CBT programs used by the patient at home (iCBT), programs that involve some telecommunication with a therapist, and synchronous videoconferencing-based CBT sessions with a live therapist.[4] When an in-person CBT provider is not available, iCBT can fill an important need.

Studies have also shown the efficacy of videoconferencing-based CBT for obsessive-compulsive disorder, as compared with alternatives such as self-help books and wait lists for in-person providers.[4] One small study of young adults randomized to videoconferencing-based CBT or traditional, in-person CBT for weekly 1-hour sessions for 12 weeks and a follow-up 6 weeks after treatment showed that videoconferencing-based CBT was associated with a statistically significant decrease in depression, anxiety, and stress symptoms.[4] A recent review examining technological interventions for substance use treatment also found partial or complete

Internet-based therapy systems can lead to clinical outcomes as good as, or better than, traditional in-person substance use disorder treatments.[21]

CHALLENGES TO THE IMPLEMENTATION
OF TELEMENTAL HEALTH MODALITIES
IN RESOURCE-LIMITED SETTINGS

This section reviews existing guidelines and suggestions for the implementation of telemedicine in general and for TMH more specifically. While guidelines exist for domestic telemedicine and TMH, there are currently no guidelines in existence to address best practice for international TMH from a regulatory perspective.[22] Regulations around telemedicine and specifically TMH vary across, and even within, countries, which further complicates the ability to standardize the implementation of TMH. Still, though guidelines for the implementation of TMH are not specific to resource-limited settings, the basic groundwork they lay out can be applied to issues more specific to resource-limited settings. Later chapters specifically address the challenges of implementing TMH interventions across international borders.

Available Guidelines

Among the most comprehensive guidelines for telemedicine currently in existence are those from the American Telemedicine Association (ATA). The ATA identifies itself as "the principal organization bringing together telemedicine practitioners, health institutions, vendors, and others involved in providing remote health using telecommunications" and is composed of members from the United States and across the world.[7] This group put out two sets of guidelines and technical standards for implementing TMH, and particularly VC-TMH, the first in 2009 and the second in 2013.[6,7] Of note, these standards are intended to provide guidance to practitioners to be tailored to particular clinical situations.[7]

An older set of guidelines also addresses the implementation of TMH more specifically. In 2001, the International Society for Mental Health Online (ISMHO) and the Psychiatric Society for Informatics (PSI) released a set of guidelines for providers of online mental health services.[2] While technology has changed significantly in the years since the publication of this set of guidelines, the principles themselves are still largely applicable to VC-TMH and other TMH encounters. Additionally, we can glean insights from these guidelines for implementing TMH services in resource-constrained settings with limited access to technology throughout the world.

In general, while these guidelines mainly address the implementation of VC-TMH in the setting of the United States, they can provide insights into the resources needed and challenges faced when setting up VC-TMH in a global setting. Each of these guidelines is referenced in the following discussion of considerations for TMH implementation.

Technical Concerns

Technical issues are also of concern when setting up VC-TMH systems internationally. For starters, even the basic technological requirements underlying VC-TMH, including a stable power source and land-based telephone or Internet service, may not be available in rural areas of the world that are the most underserved in medical and psychiatric services, where VC-TMH may be most beneficial.[12,19]

If a connection can be made, videoconferencing systems must be compatible between the patient and provider's electronic systems. The International Telecommunications Union, a specialized agency of the United Nations, has set international telecommunications standards; the use of equipment based on these standards can help to ensure successful interoperability of videoconferencing between patient and provider, regardless of platform or hardware manufacturer.[6]

Once connected, as discussed earlier in the chapter, connection speed is particularly important for analysis of a patient's movement and affect and of the provider's affect in the case of psychotherapy. While higher-speed networks allow for better visualization of patient and provider, higher-speed networks unfortunately may be less likely to be available in areas with greater need for VC-TMH, notably more rural regions.[16] Alternatively, other modalities such as store-and-forward or mobile health (mHealth) can be considered for implementation in areas where high-speed Internet is not available.

More generally, given the fallibility of all technology, it is important for the provider to lay out a technical backup plan at the initiation of treatment in VC-TMH in case of technology failure during a videoconferencing session.[7] Such a plan may include telephone-based technology troubleshooting between patient and provider or completing a session by alternate means, including over the telephone or with another on-site mental health provider.[7] Devising such a plan in advance of technical difficulties can help to make communication clear between patient and provider and to improve the therapeutic alliance.

Infrastructure Concerns

Before implementing a VC-TMH system, infrastructure must be evaluated in both the local patient or provider site and the remote provider site. A needs assessment must consider the availability of emergency resources; accessibility to labs, pharmacies, and prescription-writing capabilities on the part of the local or remote provider; and the presence of local stakeholders.[6] It is important to understand the emergency management systems available to patients who are not located at a facility with clinical staff available, including emergency room, police intervention, and the possibility of a local healthcare provider, particularly if the patient relocates over the course of treatment.[2,7]

As in all fields of medicine, financial constraints can limit the availability of TMH resources. Financially, videoconferencing equipment must be available or able to be purchased in both locations and, once installed, must be able to be kept adequately physically and electronically secure.[6]

While VC-TMH may overall be cost-effective, one deterrent to setting up a VC-TMH service is the start-up cost of current electronics, particularly of the systems that allow transmission between patient and provider to occur.[1,7] On the other hand, the savings of transport costs and ability to access patients in remote areas may make VC-TMH a worthwhile financial investment.[12] These complex forces, which play out differently in different settings, have led to inconclusive evidence regarding the cost-effectiveness of TMH interventions.[12] Work remains to be done on this topic, and costs and benefits must be considered in each particular instance of TMH implementation. A comparative analysis for cost-effectiveness of other modalities of TMH such as store-and-forward or mHealth can provide better insight into implementation strategies in different countries with different infrastructural landscapes.

Privacy Concerns

Once TMH is implemented, several steps should be undertaken to maintain patient privacy while it is in use. In general, whenever security measures are in place, the patient should be well informed of the safeguards taken to protect their health information; providers should also help patients to understand steps to take to protect their health information on the patient end.[2]

Upon initiating a TMH encounter with a patient, it is important for patient and provider alike to identify themselves, much as would be done in a live patient encounter. The ATA guidelines recommend that whereas identity verification can take place at the remote health institution if the patient is at one, when a patient is at home or otherwise in a setting without a mental health professional, the remote provider may ask the patient for further identification, including by presenting a government ID to the camera.[7] Similarly, the provider should detail to the patient his or her qualifications, licensure information, registration information, and phone numbers or web page URLs that the patient can use to verify the information.[2,7]

As in any live patient encounter, it is important that the provider document any VC-TMH encounter via paper or electronic medical record, following any applicable laws and regulations.[7] It is also important to be explicit about the use of VC in the patient encounter documentation.

Freely accessible video software may have capability, and even default settings, to allow notification to all users on a contact list about log-ons from other members of the list, to allow video "chat rooms" that can be open to other users, and to allow multiple concurrent video sessions to be initiated.[7] To protect patient confidentiality, it is imperative that such features be disabled on any video software that is used for VC-TMH.[7]

Care must also be taken to protect providers' computers from hacking, including keeping computer antivirus software up to date, ensuring the most recent security patches and updates have been installed on personal computer operating systems and videoconferencing equipment, and installing a computer firewall.[7]

Computer and mobile device encryption is also key to ensuring secure transmission of audio and video communication during a VC-TMH session.[7] Governments may develop encryption standards, such as the US Federal Information Processing Standard (FIPS 140-2) to delineate acceptable security.[7] Mobile device and portable personal computer use in VC-TMH requires additional steps to ensure security, including restriction of any stored patient contact information, access codes, the use of a timeout and reauthentication period, and software to remotely disable the device if lost or stolen.[7]

Storage of a recorded VC-TMH session or any other patient protected health information (PHI) also poses a privacy risk. Storage of such recordings is most safe on the patient's own computer, on the provider's computer only if adequate whole disk encryption has been implemented, or at a secure third-party location.[7]

In addition to patient privacy concerns, provider privacy must also be taken into consideration. The ATA guidelines recommend that videoconferencing software have capability for blocking the provider's caller information.[7] By the same token, the ISMHO/PSI guidelines note that providers may reserve the right to restrict the use of any recordings that the patient may make of their encounters.[2]

Regulatory and Legislative Concerns

Licensing laws must be followed where the provider is located and where the patient is located when care is provided, which may or may not be where the patient lives.[2,7] For this reason, it is imperative when using VC-TMH services for the provider and patient to verify, and for the provider to document, where they are located at the time of the session.[7] States and countries may have varying laws of regulatory authority and patient privacy, particularly for mental healthcare, which may allow for broader patient rights than in other specialties; as such, it is particularly crucial for the provider to be aware of all laws both in the region where the provider is practicing and where the patient is located.[6] Similarly, reimbursement may be related to where the provider and/or patient are located during a VC-TMH interaction; as such, the laws and regulations guiding provider payment must be considered when setting up a VC-TMH system.[7]

Emergency management, mandatory reporting guidelines, civil commitment laws, and any other ethical requirements to which the provider may be bound while providing care via videoconferencing must be followed for the location at which the patient is receiving care, regardless of where the patient lives.[6,7] For instance, in cases in which the patient is receiving care remotely at the site of an accredited health center, the law and licensing regulations in the region of that center should apply.[7]

Logistical Concerns

As with any clinical encounter, it is imperative to lay out expectations for patients at the initiation of any TMH encounter, particularly because TMH procedures may be unfamiliar to many patients. Additionally, it is vital for the provider to discuss expectations for contact between

VC-TMH sessions, including emergency procedures as applicable.[7] It is worthwhile, when possible, to develop a patient safety contract to prevent self-harm between sessions.[1] In the case of asynchronous communications, scheduling and turnaround time should also be laid out in advance.[2]

When implementing TMH in resource-limited settings and resource-rich settings alike, it is imperative that the practitioner have a cultural understanding of the patient population, wherever the patient might be. When working with patients from other regions and countries, it is important to consider cultural differences in body language and eye contact that may lead to differing interpretation in the immediate VC-TMH encounter, to understand cultural norms for emotional regulation, and to have a full sense of the cultural influences that may be at play in the patient's mental illness.[6] Without a good understanding of the patient's culture, the provider may inaccurately assess and diagnose the remote patient.[6]

REFERENCES

1. Deslich S, Stec B, Tomblin S, Coustasse A. Telepsychiatry in the 21(st) century: transforming healthcare with technology. Perspectives in health information management/AHIMA, American Health Information Management Association. 2013;10:1f.
2. Hsiung RC. Suggested principles of professional ethics for the online provision of mental health services. Telemedicine Journal and e-Health. 2001;7(1):39–45.
3. Norman S. The use of telemedicine in psychiatry. Journal of Psychiatric and Mental Health Nursing. 2006;13(6):771–777.
4. Aboujaoude E, Salame W, Naim L. Telemental health: a status update. World Psychiatry. 2015;14(2):223–230.
5. Neufeld JD, Yellowlees PM, Hilty DM, Cobb H, Bourgeois JA. The e-Mental Health Consultation Service: providing enhanced primary-care mental health services through telemedicine. Psychosomatics. 2007;48(2):135–141.
6. Yellowlees P, Shore J, Roberts L, American Telemedicine A. Practice guidelines for videoconferencing-based telemental health—October 2009. Telemed J E Health. 2010;16(10):1074–1089.
7. Turvey C, Coleman M, Dennison O, et al. ATA practice guidelines for video-based online mental health services. Telemed J E Health. 2013;19(9):722–730.
8. Sharp IR, Kobak KA, Osman DA. The use of videoconferencing with patients with psychosis: a review of the literature. Ann Gen Psychiatry. 2011;10(1):14.

9. Shore JH, Savin DM, Novins D, Manson SM. Cultural aspects of telepsychiatry. Journal of Telemedicine and Telecare. 2006;12(3):116–121.
10. Bidargaddi N, Schrader G, Roeger L, Bassal A, Jones L, Strobel J. Early effects of upgrading to a high bandwidth digital network for telepsychiatry assessments in rural South Australia. J Telemed Telecare. 2015;21(3):174–175.
11. Hyler SE, Gangure DP, Batchelder ST. Can telepsychiatry replace in-person psychiatric assessments? A review and meta-analysis of comparison studies. CNS Spectrums. 2005;10(5):403–413.
12. Conn D, Gajaria A, Madan R. Telepsychiatry: effectiveness and feasibility. Smart Homecare Technology and TeleHealth. 2013;2015(3):59–67.
13. Godleski L, Darkins A, Peters J. Outcomes of 98,609 U.S. Department of Veterans Affairs patients enrolled in telemental health services, 2006–2010. Psychiatric Services. 2012;63(4):383–385.
14. Garcia-Lizana F, Munoz-Mayorga I. What about telepsychiatry? A systematic review. Primary Care Companion to the Journal of Clinical Psychiatry. 2010;12(2).
15. Shore JH, Mishkind MC, Bernard J, et al. A lexicon of assessment and outcome measures for telemental health. Telemed J E Health. 2014;20(3):282–292.
16. Yellowlees PM, Odor A, Parish MB, Iosif AM, Haught K, Hilty D. A feasibility study of the use of asynchronous telepsychiatry for psychiatric consultations. Psychiatric Services. 2010;61(8):838–840.
17. Yellowlees PM, Odor A, Iosif AM, et al. Transcultural psychiatry made simple: asynchronous telepsychiatry as an approach to providing culturally relevant care. Telemed J E Health. 2013;19(4):259–264.
18. Butler TN, Yellowlees P. Cost analysis of store-and-forward telepsychiatry as a consultation model for primary care. Telemed J E Health. 2012;18(1):74–77.
19. Mars M. Telepsychiatry in Africa: a way forward? African Journal of Psychiatry. 2012;15(4):215, 217.
20. Donker T, Petrie K, Proudfoot J, Clarke J, Birch MR, Christensen H. Smartphones for smarter delivery of mental health programs: a systematic review. Journal of Medical Internet Research. 2013;15(11):e247.
21. Marsch LA, Dallery J. Advances in the psychosocial treatment of addiction: the role of technology in the delivery of evidence-based psychosocial treatment. Psychiatr Clin North Am. 2012;35(2):481–493.
22. Jefee Bahloul HMN. International telepsychiatry: a review of what has been published. Journal of Telemedicine and Telecare. 2013;19(5):293–294.

3

Telemental Health in Africa

SINCLAIR WYNCHANK AND DORA WYNCHANK

Good mental health (MH) is a necessity for all societies. Yet in almost all African countries, about 80% of those with severe MH disorders receive no treatment.[1] Telemental health (TMH) has the potential to improve this situation where MH care has been frequently neglected in the past. Other cost-effective public health strategies and interventions already exist to promote, protect, and restore MH.[2] Healthcare specialists are few in many African nations. As an extreme example, Chad has a population of 12 million, a per capita annual income of $US1,053, and a single psychiatrist.[3,4]

Telemental health uses telecommunications and information technology to aid provision of MH services. Telemental health can support individual MH providers, MH services supplied by the state, individual patients, the community, groups, or researchers. Costs of technology, which is the backbone of TMH, have steadily decreased over the last few decades, while the power of its necessary computer and communications equipment has increased. These trends will probably continue. Telemental health has had a long history in telemedicine. At the University of Nebraska in the 1950s, a two-way closed-circuit television system was used for educational and medical purposes, mainly in psychiatry. In 1973, the term "telepsychiatry" was first used to describe consultation services provided from the Massachusetts General Hospital to a medical site in Boston.[5] Telepsychiatry is one of the most widely used forms of telemedicine after teleradiology.[6]

Participants in TMH can be at two or more locations, separated by any distance. Contact between them may use various means described later, but often videoconferencing (VC). Initial uptake of TMH was slow because of psychiatry's strong associations with one-on-one interactions. Especially in sub-Saharan Africa, the requirement to speak the patient's language and associated costs and limitations of the necessary equipment and bandwidth had all contributed to the slow uptake of TMH. In recent years, TMH use has greatly increased in well-resourced countries. This is mainly due to decreased costs, improvement in data transmission rates and storage capabilities and principally because VC proved to be as effective as face-to-face interactions for many conditions.[7] Experience gained and equipment devised in these nations have increasingly been applied to TMH in resource-limited nations, often with partnerships, usually "North–South" (i.e., between well-resourced and poorly resourced countries), but "South–South" too. Africa is currently, and may well continue to be, dependent on international support for telemedicine, and cross-border telemedicine will assist in overcoming the shortage of doctors.[6]

Introduction of a TMH program typically satisfies the need for a MH service in remote, rural regions, without resident MH providers. Existing urban infrastructure can often include high-speed data links within and between major population centers in Africa. These can facilitate urban TMH. Telemedicine can be a cost-effective and efficient mean of reducing the need for the patients or healthcare providers to travel. Although such savings are valuable, in Africa it is more important to recognize that without TMH, there would often be no MH care because of lack of human resources, poverty, and long distances to any MH provider. On the other hand, TMH has been shown to increase motivation, knowledge, and confidence from patients and providers of TMH.[8]

In sub-Saharan Africa, there is much poverty and rapid urbanization. With coexisting cultural dislocation, inadequate housing, overcrowding, noise pollution, and unemployment; MH problems are caused or worsened. Those include substance use problems, insomnia, depression, and anxiety. African health services usually lack skilled personnel, appropriate infrastructure, and funding, yet are expected to serve remote and sparsely populated regions. In Africa, many medical conditions frequently present with advanced morbidity, complicated by transportation and communication barriers, which reduce availability of adequate care. Sixty percent of Africa's population still live in rural areas.[9] For various reasons, including colonialism, humanitarian disasters, wars, population displacements, and inadequate postindependence governance, African countries are often poorly resourced and unable to supply basic MH and other healthcare. However, there are many caring nongovernmental organizations (NGOs) and governments, in wealthier nations, willing to aid in MH provision and training, frequently using TMH.

TELEMENTAL HEALTH IN AFRICA

Synchronous and asynchronous modalities of TMH are implemented in Africa. Using store-and-forward (S&F) asynchronous TMH has been shown able to provide a definitive MH diagnosis and appropriate treatment on the basis of data received from the primary healthcare (PHC) physician. It is feasible and applicable in many settings and can improve access to specialized MH services, yet it certainly cannot always replace the face-to-face or VC psychiatric interview. In addition, it can support effective initial online therapies that treat selected disorders (e.g., depression and anxiety). Furthermore, successful S&F has been reported from India, including consultation, training, research and direct patient diagnosis and management.[10] Another simple and ubiquitous technology is e-mail, which is in effect another form of S&F. African use of e-mail is rapidly increasing. It allows anonymous questions to be posed online. So consultation may potentially reach individuals with mental health issues (especially men) who do not have, or have not sought, professional help. The base from which Internet usage starts is low in Africa; currently only 10.7% of households in Africa have Internet access at home, 20.7% of people use the Internet, and fixed-broadband penetration is 0.5%.[11]

Videoconferencing is the most frequently reported modality of TMH in Africa, and, importantly, African VC guidelines do exist.[12] Inexpensive TMH-VC with simple web cameras and standard Internet and computer equipment is effective and often acceptable. Many studies have demonstrated VC's effectiveness when compared with face-to-face consultations.[7] With greater availability of high-speed Internet connections, African VC use is steadily increasing. High-speed radio telecommunications and fiber-optic links, typical of technically advanced countries, are now increasingly available in Africa, usually within and between major centers. Communications at all levels of data-transfer rates are also used in Africa. Even simple VC systems can provide training in rural healthcare and successful campaigns reducing stigma associated with mental disorders. Such a pressing need to reduce such stigma in Uganda has caused measures to be introduced, described later.[3] A complex technology used in African TMH is a communication network that depends on a satellite link. The Indian government has made available one if its satellites for use in the Pan-African eNetwork, which is described in more detail later.[13] A novel form of VC is Audio Visual Assisted Therapy Aid for Refractory auditory hallucinations (AVATAR therapy), which is a form of psychotherapy used in psychotic disorders. Here, a patient suffering from persecutory auditory hallucinations interacts with a computerized representation of their persecutory voice (the avatar). A trained psychotherapist controls the avatar's responses to the patient, from hostile to supportive, during six 30-minute sessions. Gradually, the psychotic patient feels supported and gains a sense of greater power and control over the frequency and severity of auditory verbal hallucinations.[14]

Another very powerful modality for TMH used for research and educational activities, is the Internet. It is a reliable and inexpensive tool that can include web-based applications to serve in teaching, for example interactive learning, or a virtual psychiatric ward. A recently described Indian Internet-based decision support system has greatly aided diagnostic assessment and management for adults with MH disorders. The system uses a computer-based algorithm and is suitable for MH triage. When it was compared with assessments from a psychiatrist, it was found to be time-efficient. Also, the algorithm was reported to be able to assist in making psychiatric diagnoses.[15]

Innovations in TMH and its technology have not only come from the "North." Significant contributions from Africa have been adopted in other continents. Much of sub-Saharan Africa has leapfrogged the Global North's previous dependence on fixed-line telephony and instead moved directly to mobile telephony. The relatively high basic costs and slow installation of fixed-line telephony and rapidly falling costs of mobile telephony are principal reasons for this leapfrogging. Mobile-telephony coverage now is >90% in the most prosperous African countries and >50% in many of the poorest. Since telephony can be a useful means of supporting TMH, African TMH can benefit from high availability of mobile telephony. Many African nations (including South Africa, its wealthiest and most technically advanced country) suffer from frequent power-cuts. Also power surges are daily happenings in Nigeria (which also has about 300 outages yearly, lasting 5–8 hours[16]), in Kenya, and elsewhere in Africa. Successful inventions, such as the rugged BRCK, which is a device that aims to overcome these difficulties by supplying a full-power mode for 8 hours. It also ensures continuous Internet connectivity by ingeniously using a cell phone signal. This device is often used in locations without any grid electricity, so for effective TMH, (and other usage) in remote areas, this small, robust device is most useful.[16]

Africa's Telemental Health Needs

In many African nations local appreciation for the need and value of MH services is lacking. Of Togo it has been harshly said, "The majority of doctors and decision-makers in the health sector are convinced that mental illnesses are most of the time incurable and, in any case, irresponsive to classical medical protocols."[17] Such attitudes are also found in other African nations. This indicates an urgent need for educational MH activity. Telemental health programs in Africa must work toward supplying basic MH services, after the necessary training and education of PHC providers and other healthcare workers.

Africa has suffered multiple large-scale tragedies and disasters, resulting in a high burden of MH and other comorbidities. This situation is faced in several ways. Sometimes well-meaning foreigners arrive and work toward reduction of MH suffering, because of a lack of appropriate local postdisaster psychosocial expertise. But the MH disaster response may depend on precarious external initiatives and funding.[4] After a disaster, caring donors usually react swiftly, but their aid is normally short-term. After the foreigners' departure, the initial problems may return and persist.

The MH care in Africa is often based on traditional Western psychiatry, with very few psychiatrists available. Yet in Africa, traditional healers can have an important role in healthcare, whether in rural or urban settings. Any TMH interventions should perhaps link with local resources, such as traditional healers. There is great need to set up sustainable systems and services to provide adequate MH care. Telemental health systems may provide this sustainability.[4] It is always important to involve the members of the community when establishing TMH and if possible, such initiatives should be community driven.

How Other Telemental Health Experience
Can Be Useful for Africa

When implementing TMH programs in Africa, MH care providers and telecommunications equipment are needed, but that is not enough. Equally important are the necessary administrative staff and backup technical support to ensure program sustainability.[18] There have been failed telemedicine programs in Africa (e.g., in South Africa) because of these deficiencies. Notwithstanding these deficiencies, TMH models in high-income countries are often applicable to Africa. This process has many levels. Initially, major medical centers provide amenities for distant rural telecommunities. Next, further services are established, including chronic illness management and crisis interventions for poorly served populations. Ongoing consultations can then serve as means to provide capacity building for local healthcare workers. The potential of TMH has been recognized for several decades, yet its uptake has been slow (in all types of societies) for several reasons, including general reluctance to adopt new methods and technology.[19] A little-appreciated necessity for successful TMH is to recognize and encourage a local "champion," and several reports indicate its importance.[20]

AFRICA'S CURRENT TELEMENTAL HEALTH

Several "North–South" collaborative TMH projects are underway in Africa.

Cameroon

Cameroon, a nation of 22 million population, has only seven registered psychiatrists. A Swiss–Cameroonian TMH collaboration, involving the Cameroonian Ministry of Public Health, the University Hospital of Geneva, and the Nant Foundation,[21] serves Cameroon's dire MH needs. These Swiss participants also aid the MH of other francophone nations. The collaboration trains PHC providers to identify MH issues and facilitate access to appropriate psychopharmacological interventions. Primary healthcare providers must collaboratively be able to provide culturally sensitive care to this underserved population. Regrettably, much current attention to MH care in Africa is concerned with trauma, because of the many wars and armed conflicts of the last few decades. Too often, this results in psychological trauma, which will be encountered by PHC practitioners. They require appropriate training, which is gradually being made available. Telemental health education, outlined here, is proving cost-effective and is steadily increasing in availability.

Uganda

The US Alderman Foundation, working with the Ugandan Ministry of Health in a private-public partnership, expressed cautious optimism about the effectiveness of its pilot group interventions for adults with mental distress in postconflict settings and stated that it may have considerable MH benefits. Thus, it should be extended. Telemental health is likely to prove valuable to train the MH care providers necessary to treat psychotrauma.[22]

Democratic Republic of the Congo

The Democratic Republic of the Congo has no general MH care. However, TMH infrastructure is being set up in the Uvira region, according to the Uvira Psychosocial Rehabilitation Center website.[23] No more details are available at the time of writing this chapter. This region is in great need of MH services, as it is an area of active armed conflict and war.

Ghana

Another collaboration, between Ghana, the European Union (EU), and the University of San Francisco is underway. The collaboration held a workshop at Nkoranza, Ghana, in 2015 titled, "Open Medical Record System-Based Mobile-Telepsychiatry for Community Mental-Healthcare Professionals."[24] This project will provide low-cost TMH using VC (including neuropsychiatric assessment, community-based clinical support services, culture-specific MH screening, assessment, and monitoring tools).

Somaliland

Projects initiated by Somaliland expatriate psychiatrists who live in high-income countries (Norway, Sweden, Denmark, and the UK) are supported by the latter two nations and coordinated by the Somaliland participants. Skype-mediated VC is used to provide diagnostic assessments and management of MH issues. Language and cultural barriers are bypassed by cultural-matching of providers with patients. An initial report[25] indicated feasibility of such a VC approach. The report indicated that main diagnoses seen in adult females were mood disorders, psychosis, and epilepsy and in male adults were psychosis, epilepsy, khat-induced psychosis, and mood disorders. The project was extended to include tele-education and to recruit more expatriate MH providers. This Skype-based telepsychiatry is believed by UK[25] and Somaliland[26] participants to provide an effective and inexpensive MH service. A feasible project, it represents a model for other African nations with minimal MH services, as most African nations have expatriate MH providers trained and living in high-income countries. However, some have voiced concerns over data security and privacy when using voice-over Internet protocols like Skype.[27]

Kenya

Another program, supported by the EU and the African MH Foundation, trains Somali doctors in Kenya to recognize MH issues, provide nonpharmacological MH interventions, and provide primary and secondary MH services. Subsequent telesupervision allows TMH continued management and training.[28]

South–South Projects

There are several "South–South" TMH projects underway. Since 2010, the Pan-African eNetwork, a large telemedical-educational service between

India and 47 African nations, has been operational. It functions with an initial budget of $US125M.[13] The necessary telecommunication uses undersea fiber-optic cables, an Indian satellite, and 169 very small aperture terminal two-way satellite dishes in Africa, and probably constitutes Africa's largest noncommercial information and computer technology network. This service is funded by the Indian government and is intended to aid provision of African health services. A large majority of sub-Saharan African nations participate. Their academic institutions ensure that appropriate staff members receive instruction, present cases, and discuss problems during the daily VC sessions.

Cross-Cultural Telemental Health

African nations are often multicultural, so the different cultural backgrounds of patient and TMH healthcare worker may cause difficulties. With the large population movements worldwide during the last half-century, such difficulties have been experienced in most nations. Much has been written on cross-cultural telepsychiatry, for culture differences between practitioner and patient are even more important here than in most other medical disciplines. In Africa, a typical TMH provider is a city dweller. If the patient is from a remote rural region, the provider's ignorance of rural culture may cause less effective interactions. One Danish cross-cultural study investigated 52 patients who spoke 9 languages, but only culturally matched MH care providers were used. (Interpreters obtained only informed consent and initiated the study.) The patients were generally very satisfied with the telepsychiatry, being willing to recommend TMH to others and to repeat it for themselves. Unsurprisingly, they preferred their own language for the interaction, rather than a translator.[29] Such cross-cultural TMH has been reported in the United States using S&F interactions between providers and their Spanish-speaking patients whose words are translated into English. Here, this method was deemed feasible and able to provide general diagnostic reliability.[30] Another cultural barrier, frequently encountered in rural Africa, is discomfort with modern technology, particularly among older persons. In cultures where personal relationships are of great significance, TMH is perceived as an impersonal interaction. In spite of some difficulties encountered in cross-cultural and cross-generational TMH, it may well be feasible in culturally diverse Africa.

Telemental Health Education

The Pan-African eNetwork, mentioned previously, has provided over 600 courses to date. Almost all are in English, with a few in French. The courses are prepared and delivered by members of leading Indian educational institutions and universities. Mostly they deal with nonpsychiatric medical topics, but childhood ADHD, anxiety, stress, and the mental status examination have been included. There are daily medical teleconsultations in all disciplines.

Another enterprising form of TMH education is to use the broadcast media, and this has created awareness and aided provision of support systems for those needing MH services in Nigerian rural and urban centers.[31] Such success deserves replication elsewhere in Africa. The South African Depression and Anxiety Group was established in 1995 and produces "Mental Health Matters," a daily television talk-show that discusses MH issues including anxiety, depression, exam stress, bullying, substance abuse, trauma, bipolar, suicide prevention, and self-mutilation. About 4 million South Africans watch it in addition to viewers in 49 other African countries, principally Kenya, Mauritius, Nigeria, Tanzania, and Uganda. The show targets youth, young adults, and parents to discuss MH issues encountered daily. Participants include patients, psychiatrists, psychologists, and general practitioners. The TV program is supported by a toll-free helpline, with its number aired during and after every program, allowing contact with free telephonic counselors, who provide information, self-help tips, support, and referrals to resources in the caller's area. Further support is found on a large website and free multilingual brochures on MH issues, including depression, bipolar, post-traumatic stress disorder, obsessive-compulsive

disorder, anxiety, trauma, sleeping disorders, schizophrenia, teen suicide, and substance abuse. Workshops and training programs are directed
toward commercial companies, educational establishments, clinics, youth
groups, correctional facilities, and traditional healers (personal communication, J. Ilondo, September 16, 2015).

The value of PHC providers aiding MH care is well established and effective, even when the patient may not make optimal progress.[32] Telemental
health education programs are underway, for example in Uganda.[3] This
educational plan is to establish MH units in 13 regional hospitals throughout the country to train PHC providers to offer basic MH care.[3] In African
MH provision, patients usually choose to present in primary care settings
for their psychological symptoms, due in part to stigma related to psychiatric clinics. With appropriate training, primary care providers diagnose,
manage, and refer patients who do not respond (or those who present
with complex MH issues).

Telemental health education should not only be directed toward MH
providers. Patients and lay healthcare workers can also benefit in regions
that lack MH facilities. For example, in schizophrenia, even simple telephonic follow-up, following psychoeducation in the clinic, decreases caregiver burden and depressive symptoms and supports home-based care.[33]
In Uganda, TMH education has been taken further, with moves underway
for the government to provide MH education for schoolgoers.[34] Important
aspects of community psychoeducation are destigmatization of mental illness and encouragement to receive effective MH services. Too often in
Africa, barriers include the long distance to a MH care facility. Advantages
of TMH are evident. Beneficiaries of MH services are the patient's family
and community.

The advantages of TMH are also apparent in training schemes for psychiatrists and other MH care workers worldwide. Some experience of
TMH should be included in all training, and slowly this is being done.
Telemental health training typically includes supervised provision of clinical care and even didactic teaching and awareness of aspects of medicolegal and cross-cultural perspectives.[35] When training MH workers on
early intervention in psychosis, VC-based education was found to be as

effective as face-to-face interactions. In countries, such as South Africa, where healthcare graduates must perform 2 years' community service after graduation, TMH can facilitate this work. New graduates are much more likely to use TMH in their later work.

Legal and Ethical Aspects of Telemental Health

The electronic transmission of sensitive data when implementing TMH can result in loss of confidentiality and privacy, in ways different from conventional MH care. Secure transmission, password protection, and data encryption can all help to reduce such losses and are relatively easy to install and use. Although malpractice considerations are not common in Africa, they do occur in some settings. Recordings of VC sessions can be retained and this may discourage potential malpractice suits. There is potential lack of confidentiality and privacy if data passes through a telecommunications network. Electronic transmission of data can be both an advantage and disadvantage. In planning stages of any TMH intervention, appropriate attention should be paid to data security. However, there is virtually no current legislation relevant to TMH extant and none in African countries. But the question has been discussed in South Africa. Existing legal provisions applicable to MH are often old-fashioned and in need of revision.[36] When new MH legislation is drawn up, TMH must be taken into account.

A basic premise for ethical TMH practice is to consider the patient a person, even if face-to-face contact is never made with the MH provider. In order for the patient (and the MH providers) to be fully protected there must be appropriate measures to ensure confidentiality, privacy, informed consent, security, practitioner credentialing, equity of access, and promoting independence versus dependency. With its third-party involvement, forensic psychiatry introduces additional ethical considerations.

Little has been written about African forensic TMH, but programs have been deemed feasible.[37] These applications of TMH can help provide courts with pretrial assessments of those with possible mental disorders and offer psycho–tele-education about MH issues to the legal sector. Telemental health is suitable in situations where safety is a concern, as VC can provide ability to make the assessment without physical risk for the forensic psychiatrist. Forensic TMH obviates much travel, and prisoners tend to have no preference between TMH and face-to-face-interactions. Another advantage of TMH is to reduce waiting periods for MH assessments where urgent evaluation is needed.

Much political enthusiasm has been expressed for extension of TMH in different African countries (with Archbishop Tutu among the proponents). However, this is usually accompanied by regrets that the health services have insufficient resources. The demonstration of successful "North–South" and other TMH projects may reinforce the enthusiasm. Confirmation of their cost-effectiveness and greatly improved MH care provision in regions previously without any such services, may convince politicians to adopt more TMH.

The Future

The future of African TMH is to employ this powerful modality in aiding primary care providers in a decentralized manner. In many sub-Saharan nations, there is urgent need to address marginalization of MH disorders, the high levels of stigma, and gross deficiency in the provision of MH care. Telemental health can be a useful tool in redressing this deficiency as it is generally acknowledged as a valuable and cost-effective alternative to face-to-face conventional MH services. As new programs are set up they should have rigorous evaluation assessments built into them, wherever possible. This would increase the direct proven empirical evidence of such cost-effectiveness by formal evaluation. Future African TMH should build on, extend, or duplicate previous relevant successes, such as the Somaliland expatriate project. Indeed, plans are underway for this project to include all major Somaliland cities and appropriate educational programs.[26] The successful uses of broadcast media in Nigeria and

South Africa to aid creation of awareness and to provide support systems for those needing MH care in both rural and urban settings[31] should be recognized as examples of inexpensive and effective TMH educational measures.

The future of TMH in Africa should address the existing serious shortage in MH services by improving access to better-quality care. Second opinions can be given by experts where cases are complex and treating healthcare professionals need support.[38] Above all, it should build on the successful work outlined, using practical, proven means, coupled with quantitative, formal evaluation. African MH care, appropriately embracing TMH, will provide increased benefits for those in greatest need. This will achieve a crucial component of the World Health Organization's aim to ensure good health: "A state of complete physical, mental and social well-being" and not just the absence of (mental) illness.

REFERENCES

1. World Health Organization. Mental health action plan 2013–2020. World Health Organization, Geneva, Switzerland. http://www.who.int/mental_health/publications/action_plan/en/. Published 2013. Accessed July 4, 2015.
2. World Health Organization. Mental health: strengthening our response 2014. World Health Organization, Geneva, Switzerland. http://www.who.int/mediacentre/factsheets/fs220/en/. Published August, 2014. Accessed July 4, 2015.
3. World Health Organization. Mental health atlas 2011. World Health Organization, Geneva, Switzerland. http://www.who.int/mediacentre/multimedia/podcasts/2011/mental_health_17102011/en/. Published October 19, 2011. Accessed July 4, 2015.
4. Elmasri M. Mental health beyond the crises. Bull WHO. 2011;89:326–327.
5. Myers K, Cain S. Work Group on Quality Issues. Bernet W, Bukstein O, Walter H, et al. Practice parameter for telepsychiatry with children and adolescents. Journal of the American Academy of Child and Adolescent Psychiatry. 2008;47(12):1468–1483.
6. Mars, M. Guest editorial: Telepsychiatry in Africa: a way forward? African Journal of Psychiatry (Johannesbg). 2012;15(4):215–217.
7. García-Lizana F, Muñoz-Mayorga I. What about telepsychiatry? A systematic review. Primary Care Companion to the Journal of Clinical Psychiatry. 2010;12(2):2.

8. Adler G, Pritchett LR, Kauth MR, Nadorff D. A pilot project to improve access to telepsychotherapy at rural clinics. Journal of Telemed and E-Health. 2014;20(1):83–85.

9. World Urbanization Prospects, the 2011 Revision. United Nations, Department of Economic and Social Affairs, Population Division. New York: United Nations. 2012.

10. Malhotra S, Chakrabarti S, Shah R. Telepsychiatry: promise, potential, and challenges. Indian Journal of Psychiatry. 2013;55(1):3–11.

11. The World in 2013, ICT facts and figures. International Telecommunications Union. http://www.itu.int/en/ITU-D/Statistics/Documents/facts/ICTFactsFigures2015.pdf. Published May 2015. Accessed September 16, 2015.

12. Chipps J, Ramlall S, Mars M. Practice guidelines for videoconference-based telepsychiatry in South Africa. African Journal of Psychiatry (Johannesbg). 2012;15(4):271–282.

13. Pan African e-Network Project 2015. http://www.apollotelehealth.com:9013/ATNF/panAfricanProject.jsp. Published September 16, 2004. Accessed July 4, 2015.

14. Leff J, Williams G, Huckvale M, Arbuthnot M, Leff AP. Avatar therapy for persecutory auditory hallucinations: what is it and how does it work? Psychosis. 2014;6(2):166–176.

15. Malhotra S, Chakrabarti S, Shah R, et al. Development of a novel diagnostic system for a telepsychiatric application: a pilot validation study. BMC Research Notes. 2014;7:508.

16. Jackson T. BRCK could bring a reliable Internet connection to some of the most remote parts of Africa. http://thenextweb.com/gadgets/2014/07/16/brck-africa-funding/. Published July 16, 2014. Accessed July 4, 2015.

17. Togo: Setting up Community Mental Health Care, Foundation d'Harcourt, 2015. http://www.fondationdharcourt.org/the-projects/togo-setting-up-community-mental-health-care. Published 2015. Accessed July 4, 2015.

18. Chipps J, Ramlall S, Madigoe T, King H, Mars M. Developing telepsychiatry services in KwaZulu-Natal: an action research study. African Journal of Psychiatry (Johannesbg). 2012;15(4):255–263.

19. Myers KM, Valentine JM, Melzer SM. Feasibility, acceptability, and sustainability of telepsychiatry for children and adolescents. Psychiatric Services. 2007;58(11):1493–1496.

20. Pepler A, Boydell KM, Teshima J, Volpe T, Braunberger PG, Minden D. Transforming Child and Youth Mental Health Care via Innovative Technological Solutions. Healthc Q. 2011;14(Spec No):92–102.

21. Helina—Health Informatics in Africa 2014. http://archive-org.com/org/h/helina-online.org/2014-04-04_3897880_2/Programm_HELINA_HEALTH_INFORMATICS_IN_AFRICA/. Published April 4, 2014. Accessed July 4, 2015.

22. Nakimuli-Mpungu E, Okello J, Kinyanda E, et al. The impact of group counseling on depression, post-traumatic stress and function outcomes: a prospective comparison study in the Peter C. Alderman trauma clinics in northern Uganda. Journal of Affective Disorders. 2013;151(1):78–84.

23. Experimenting with telepsychiatry in East Congo. Centre de Réadaptation Psycho-Social d'Uvira (CRPU). http://www.crpduvira.org/Pages/ExperimentingwithTelepsychiatryinEastCongo.aspx. Published January 30, 2014. Accessed July 4, 2015.

24. Awakame J. Inauguration of the West African Centre for Health Informatics 2014. https://talk.openmrs.org/t/inauguration-of-the-west-african-centre-for-health-informatics/453. Published July 1, 2014. Accessed July 4, 2015.

25. Abdi YA, Elmi JY. Internet based telepsychiatry: a pilot case in Somaliland. Medicine, Conflict, and Survival. 2011;27(3):145–150.

26. Syed Sheriff RJ, Baraco AF, Nour A. Public-academic partnerships: improving human resource provision for mental health in Somaliland. Psychiatric Services. 2010;61(3):225–227.

27. Mars M. Telemedicine and advances in urban and rural healthcare delivery in Africa. Progress in Cardiovascular Diseases. 2013;56(3):326–335.

28. Ndetei DM. Tele-psychiatry between Nairobi and Somalia, Royal College of Psychiatrists, Quarterly Newsletter—African International Division. 2010;3(5):12–13.

29. Mucic D. Transcultural telepsychiatry and its impact on patient satisfaction, Journal of Telemedicine and Telecare. 2010;16(5):237–242.

30. Yellowlees PM, Odor A, Iosif AM. Transcultural psychiatry made simple: asynchronous telepsychiatry as an approach to providing culturally relevant care. Journal of Telemedicince and E-Health. 2013;19(4):259–264.

31. Omoera OS, Aihevba P. Broadcast media intervention in mental health challenge. Antrocom Online Journal of Anthropology 2012;8:439–452.

32. Myers KM, Lieberman D. Telemental health: responding to mandates for reform in primary healthcare. Journal of Telemedicine andE-Health. 2013;19(6):438–443.

33. Ozkan B, Erdem E, Demirel Ozsoy S, Zararsiz G. Effect of psychoeducation and telepsychiatric follow up given to the caregiver of the schizophrenic patient on family burden, depression and expression of emotion, Pakistan Journal of Medical Sciences. 2013;29(5):1122–1127.

34. Liebling, H, Davidson L, Akello FG, Ochola G. Improvements to national health policy: mental health, mental health bill, legislation and justice. African Journal of Traumatic Stress. 2014;3(2):55–63.

35. Sunderji N, Crawford A, Jovanovic M. Telepsychiatry in graduate medical education: a narrative review. Journal of Academic Psychiatry. 2015;39(1):55–62.

36. Glover JA, Williams E, Hazlett LJ, Campbell N. Connecting to the future: telepsychiatry in postgraduate medical education. Journal of Telemedicine and E-health. 2013;19(6):474–479.

37. Mars M, Ramlall S, Kaliski S. Forensic telepsychiatry: a possible solution for South Africa? African Journal of Psychiatry (Johannesbg). 2012;15(4):244–247.

38. Gruber HG, Wolf B, Reiher M. Status, barriers and potential of telemedical systems in African countries. AFRICON, 2011, IEEE, 2011. http://ieeexplore.ieee.org/xpl/articleDetails.jsp?arnumber=6072022&filter%3DAND%28p_IS_Number%3A6071956%29%26rowsPerPage%3D100. Published September 2011. Accessed September 16, 2015.

4

Telemental Health in South Africa

MAURICE MARS

South Africa was an early leader in telemedicine on the African continent, but telemedicine stagnated for nearly 10 years after failure of a National Telemedicine System. The need for telemental health services in South Africa has been identified in two reviews, and a fledgling service has begun.[1,2] With the government's vision of providing all South Africans with access to quality healthcare through National Health Insurance, there is renewed interest in telemedicine. The opportunity exists to expand on the steps already taken toward telemental health services.

BACKGROUND

South Africa is a large and diverse nation with a population of 54 million people, of whom approximately a third live in rural areas.[3] It is a constitutional democracy and is divided into nine provinces with 11 official languages. Its population is young: the median age of 26.5 years, and 30% of the population is under 15 years of age. While considered an upper-middle-income country with a GDP of US$366 billion, it is a country of great inequality, with a GINI coefficient of 63.[4,5] Approximately 25% of those of working age are unemployed, and 77% of the rural population live below the national poverty line.

BURDEN OF DISEASE

South Africa faces a quadruple burden of disease, HIV/AIDS and tuberculosis (TB), high rates of maternal and child morbidity, injury and violence, and an increase in noncommunicable diseases. Initial denial by the government that HIV causes AIDS has resulted in 6.3 million people living with AIDS in South Africa, more than any other country, with 80% of those eligible currently on antiretroviral therapy. The HIV prevalence nationally is 10.2%, and 19.1% among 15- to 49-year-olds.[6] In KwaZulu-Natal between 40% and 60% of pregnant women are HIV positive.[7] Those infected with HIV have a high prevalence of mental illness at 43.7% compared with the general population at 16.5%. Tuberculosis is a comorbidity of HIV/AIDS and its incidence and prevalence is high, 860 and 715 per 100,000 people, respectively. Multiple-drug-resistant TB and extremely drug-resistant TB are on the rise. Comorbid mental disorders of HIV and TB are associated with high-risk behavior, poor treatment adherence, and inability to access care.

In one province, 47% of pregnant women were diagnosed with antenatal depression.[8] Violence is endemic: The homicide rate is 35.7 per 100,000 people.[6] A 1997 study found that 23% of people between the ages of 16 and 64 had been exposed to one or more violent event, and of these people, 78% have one or more symptoms of post-traumatic stress disorder.[9] In addition, South Africa has major challenges with substance abuse and the highest incidence of alcohol abuse in the world after Ukraine, further fueling crime and violence.[6] All of these add to the burden of mental health disorders.

HEALTH SYSTEM

There are parallel healthcare systems in South Africa, a state-subsidized public sector and a private commercial sector. The government spends 8.9% of the GDP on health. Budgets and provision of health services in the public sector are devolved to the nine provincial Departments of Health. The public sector serves 84% of the population in primary health clinics (PHCs) and district, regional, tertiary, and quaternary hospitals. The remaining 16% of the population uses the private sector and is covered by self-funded insurance or pays directly out of pocket.[3] The per capita health spending in the private sector is 10 times that of the public sector.[10]

While South Africa is reported to have 78 doctors per 100,000 people,[11] it is estimated that the actual number of doctors actively practicing in the country is nearer 55 per 100,000.[12] There is a shortage of doctors in public-sector general hospitals, with an estimated 49% of all medical practitioner posts in public hospitals unfilled in 2010. The situation remains largely unchanged.[3] There is a discrepancy in the reported number of psychiatrists in the country. According to the WHO statistics there are 0.39 psychiatrists per 100,000 people, which, based on a total population of 50 million people, equates to 195 psychiatrists. According to the South African Association of Psychiatrists there are 350 practicing psychiatrists in the country, 60% of whom work in the private sector.[13] This leaves approximately 140 psychiatrists serving roughly 40 million people, 0.35 psychiatrists per 100,000 people in the public sector compared with 2.1 psychiatrists per 100,000 people in the private sector. There are similar shortages of nonspecialist doctors, psychologists, nurses, and social workers in the mental health sector. Twenty-three mental hospitals provide 22.7 beds per 100,000 people with general hospitals and community residential facilities providing 2.7 and 3.5 beds per 100,000 people respectively.

Medical services are also provided by traditional healers. They are recognized by legislation, the Traditional Health Practitioners Act of 2007, and have been able to register with the Interim Traditional Practitioners Council since 2014. Approximately 60% of the population consults first or exclusively with traditional healers.[14]

Traditional healers are either diviners, herbalists, or both. Their mental health literacy is low, and their belief is that the cause of mental health disorders is either supernatural or natural. Most disorders are deemed to be supernatural and due to bewitchment. Bewitched patients present with psychotic behavior, which can only be diagnosed by a traditional healer and cured with traditional medicine. Natural mental health disorders including epilepsy and those caused by alcohol or other substance abuse are considered to be amenable to Western medicine. Approximately 50% of those with a mental disorder have consulted a traditional healer.[15]

MENTAL HEALTH POLICY AND LEGISLATION

A mental health policy was developed in 1997 but was not published for various reasons. The Mental Health Care Act (2002) promulgated in 2004 introduced substantial changes to the provision of mental healthcare in the country. Selected regional and district hospitals were designated under the Act to perform 72-hour observations of involuntary and assisted mental healthcare users with the intention of providing local access to care and reducing premature or unnecessary transfers to psychiatric hospitals. This was not supported by a dedicated budget, implementation plan, or increase in staff and facilities.[16]

The national mental health authority, the Directorate: Mental Health and Substance Abuse, advises the government on mental health policies and legislation. A Mental Health Policy Framework for South Africa and Strategic Plan 2013–2020 has been approved by the National Health Council. The major objectives of the eight-point plan are to scale up decentralized integrated primary mental health services, which include community-based, PHC, and district hospital–level care; increase public awareness regarding mental health and reduce stigma and discrimination associated with mental illness; promote the mental health of the South African population, through collaboration between the Department of Health and other sectors; empower local communities, especially mental health service users and carers, to participate in promoting mental well-being and recovery within their community; promote and protect the human rights of people living with mental illness; adopt a multisectoral approach to tackling the vicious cycle of poverty and mental ill-health; establish a monitoring and evaluation system for mental healthcare; and ensure that the planning and provision of mental health services is evidence-based.[17]

Standards and norms for mental healthcare have been developed, as have norms for people with severe psychiatric conditions; community-based mental healthcare; and child and adolescent mental health services. Few of the facility and staffing norms have been met. A recent study in KwaZulu-Natal Province found that there were only 25% of the requisite acute-care beds and 80% of forensic beds, but a substantial oversupply of long-term beds. These were served by only 25% of the number of psychiatrists and 25% of the registrars/residents and medical officers needed to comply with the standards.[18] In the absence of professional staff, the shortage of acute-care beds may be appropriate. There are limited data on funding of mental health in the nine provinces. It is acknowledged in the National Policy Framework that mental health is underfunded. Over a 5-year period, budgetary increases to psychiatric hospitals in KwaZulu-Natal were a quarter of those to general hospitals.[18]

TELEMEDICINE IN SOUTH AFRICA

South Africa has a National eHealth Strategy for the public sector, published in 2012, which aims to leverage information and communication technologies in support of a national health information system and the proposed National Health Insurance. The strategy appropriately incorporates telemedicine as a means of supporting rural patients, improving quality of care by providing access to scarce specialist skills, overcoming the shortage of doctors and nurses in rural areas, reducing unnecessary patient transfer, overcoming the sense of isolation of doctors in rural areas, providing continuing medical education, and facilitating medical research.[19]

The postapartheid government saw the potential of telemedicine. A National Telemedicine Task team was formed in 1998 and commissioned to develop a national telemedicine strategy for South Africa and implement a National Telemedicine System. After installation of infrastructure for phase one of the project at 28 sites by the National Department of Health, subsequent management and funding of the telemedicine services devolved to the relevant Provincial Department of Health, which had not budgeted for telemedicine nor provided administrative posts. A national telemedicine research center was also established at the Medical Research Council.

The project failed. The reasons were many and varied, but can be largely attributed to the top-down approach followed by lack of buy-in by the provincial Departments of Health and local clinicians. Government then withdrew financial support, and phases two and three were not implemented.[20]

Telemedicine stagnated, receiving little support from the national or provincial Departments of Health except in the Eastern Cape and Limpopo Provinces. The Medical Research Council developed several telemedicine projects in collaboration with the University of Stellenbosch. The University of KwaZulu-Natal developed clinical and educational services and telemedicine infrastructure in KwaZulu-Natal through donor funding and use of university resources. A recent survey of telemedicine in the public sector found that a third of public hospitals had telemedicine or tele-educational facilities and less than 3% of PHCs had infrastructure for telemedicine. Apart from teleradiology, tele-education, and teledermatology, there are no sustained telemedicine programs in the public sector.[21]

In the private sector, many radiology practices have adopted teleradiology, with digital images stored electronically in picture-archiving systems and accessed using radiology information systems and with the reporting radiologists not necessarily at the same site as the patient. Aspects of pathology have been automated and meet the definition of telemedicine. Doctors and nurses are sending and receiving e-mail from patients and storing patient data on computers and doctors are sending photographs from their smartphones and tablet PCs to their colleagues for second-opinion advice.[22]

TELEMEDICINE FOR MENTAL HEALTH

Telemental health and telepsychology were not considered for phase one of the National Telemedicine System. Current activity in mental health is embryonic and very limited. It can be divided into clinical support through videoconference, tele-education in mental health, and mobile phone–based initiatives aimed at improving HIV and TB treatment adherence, data gathering, screening, behavior change, and support for women during and immediately after pregnancy.

A review of telemental health outlined the potential benefits of telemental health for South Africa.[2] The need for forensic telemental health to reduce the time that prisoners spend in jail awaiting assessment of adjudicative competence in South Africa has also been highlighted and videoconference consultation has been proposed.[1]

Real-time telemental health is well established in high-income countries (HICs). The need for expensive videoconferencing equipment, adequate bandwidth, and the ability to converse in the patient's language has limited its uptake in South Africa. In most provinces there are few district hospitals with videoconferencing facilities. An alternative would be to use voice-over Internet protocols like Skype. While there are concerns over data security and privacy with Skype, simple solutions like this are needed.

There have been two published reports of videoconference-based telemental health in South Africa, both from the public sector. A telepsychology service between a nurse-led PHC in Beaufort West in the Western Cape Province and the University of the Western Cape allowed assessment of agitated patients presenting at the clinic. This was of particular benefit over weekends, when the patients would otherwise have been taken to the police cells and held until the district surgeon could see them during the week. While deemed successful, the program was short-lived because the equipment was stolen. No data on actual use are available.[23]

The second, a fledgling telemental health service, was reported in KwaZulu-Natal, where several district hospitals have videoconferencing equipment with Integrated Services Digital Network (ISDN)–based connectivity. This followed a number of studies undertaken to facilitate the implementation of telemental health in South Africa. These looked at the need for telemental health,[24] the readiness of hospitals to take part in telemental health,[25] the introduction of telemental health services at two hospitals,[26] the development of an administrative model for telemental health,[27] and the production of "Guidelines for the Practice of Telemental Health in South Africa," which were endorsed by the College of Psychiatry of South Africa.[28]

The needs analysis confirmed the shortage of psychiatrists in the region. It also provided insight into shortcomings of staff, facilities, hospital administration, and management of patients admitted for 72-hour observation.[16] The "eReadiness" study identified problems at the management level. Ten of the 11 district managers and 41 hospital managers were interviewed. The district managers were often unfamiliar with administrative issues related to telemedicine, the relevant equipment in their hospitals, telemedicine services already in place, and the plans of the provincial Department of Health for telemedicine. They were also unwilling to "provide comments for other people," despite the project having been approved by the provincial Department of Health.[25]

As part of the clinical services provided at regional hospitals, psychiatrists are expected to provide outreach services, both clinical and educational, to hospitals in their district. The sole psychiatrist at one of the regional hospitals, some 200 km away from the medical school, was required to provide services to rural district hospitals where there were no psychiatrists. He initially began by conducting follow-up consultations by videoconference with patients he had previously seen at the district hospital. As his experience and confidence in using videoconferencing grew, he began consulting new patients with a local doctor present during the consultation. The local doctor benefited from the one-to-one interaction with the psychiatrist, with time spent after each consultation discussing the patient and further management. The "telepsychiatrist" saw on average four patients per session and conducted biweekly sessions, saving him from driving to rural hospitals.

Two forms of tele-education have been reported for psychiatry. As part of an outreach service to hospitals designated to admit mental health patients for 72-hour observation, psychiatrists at the University of KwaZulu-Natal videorecorded lectures on mental health topics, which were then saved to DVD and sent to hospitals for use by staff.[27] A videoconference-based tele-education service was developed for psychiatry registrars (residents) in training. This obviated the need to travel to Durban for teaching. Over the 2 years reported, 6.5 hours of formal psychiatry teaching were broadcast each week. The savings effected by not having to travel to the medical school would have paid for the setup costs of two videoconferencing venues within 6 months.[29]

There is also need for forensic telemental services. In South Africa, pretrial detainees awaiting assessment of adjudicative competence may be held in jail for over a year before undergoing a 30-day observation. Videoconference forensic assessment has been proposed.[1]

MOBILE HEALTH (MHEALTH) FOR MENTAL HEALTH

The cellular phone provides a simple and relatively cost-effective means of transmitting data between people for health. While there are almost 100 mHealth projects that have been or are being implemented in South Africa there are few that deal specifically with mental health. Others that address drug adherence for HIV and TB, address behavioral change, and provide educational material or access to information can be considered to have potentially beneficial effects on mental health.

Project Masihambisane is a randomized controlled trial aimed at improving health and well-being of HIV-positive mothers and their babies. Mothers were required to attend four prenatal and four postnatal small-group peer-mentoring sessions run by local community health workers. Assessments were made at the first antenatal clinic visit (baseline), postpartum, and 6 and 12 months postpartum. A computerized mobile phone interview protocol was used to aid data collection and assist in maintaining data quality. Significant reduction in depressed mood between baseline and 12 months was seen in the intervention group.[30]

In Khayelitsha, a socioeconomically deprived periurban settlement in Cape Town where most people live in informal housing, community health workers confirmed the feasibility of conducting screening for perinatal depression using the 10-point Edinburgh Postnatal Depression scale as part of their outreach program. A previously validated translation of the tool in isiXhosa, the predominant language in the settlement, was programmed into a cellular phone, and the survey was administered prepartum and 12 weeks postpartum.[31]

In a randomized controlled trial (Cellphones4Africa) HIV-positive mothers were reminded to attend appointments and bring their child for HIV testing. This was shown to have a strong psychological effect on those participating. A second component of this was two-way communication with users phoning specific phone numbers linked to a specific query, and a text message answer was sent back at no cost to the user.[32]

The South African Depression and Anxiety Group is the largest mental health support and advocacy group in Africa. As an addition to its counseling call center, it has a short message service (SMS) that enables counselors to obtain contact details and telephone the person in need. It also offers a free medication reminder service with an associated free counseling service.[33]

The National Department of Health has started an initiative, MomConnect, to register every pregnant woman in South Africa by SMS. Appointment reminders and information based on the stage of pregnancy are sent by SMS up to the child's first birthday. Messages are sent out in one of five of the official languages, selected by the mother. There is an associated Web-based community portal "askmama.mobi," where more detailed information can be accessed. Several of the Web pages address postnatal depression and changes in emotion.[34]

The recently announced GSMA (Global System for Mobile Communication Association)'s Mobile for Development program aims to improve maternal and child health by making access to cellular phones and airtime more affordable. The handsets will have an embedded Smart Health application and the SIM cards will allow free access to health content and facilitate health registration and data collection.

OBSTACLES TO TELEMEDICINE
AND TELEMENTAL HEALTH IN SOUTH AFRICA

There is little doubt that there is need to improve access to mental health-care. Roughly 50% of people with mental health disorders in South Africa do not receive treatment. But who is to provide this additional care and how? Telemedicine is a potential solution but there are several issues impeding uptake of telemental healthcare in South Africa. These are mostly generic and not specific to telemental health.

Human Resources

There are not enough psychiatrists to meet the current demand, so an obvious solution is to increase the production of both doctors and sub-sequently psychiatrists. There have been no new medical schools built in the country since the mid-1970s, and although the medical schools have increased their intake, production is not keeping pace with population growth. Two new medical schools have been proposed but not yet opened. Emigration of young doctors and worse, psychiatrists, exacerbates the problem.

Videoconference-based telemental health presents a solution, but it places extra steps in the routine workflow, and requires additional techni-cal and administrative support at both the send and receive sites. For the psychiatrist in the public sector, the extra steps in the workflow are offset by the time saved by not having to drive to rural district hospitals for out-reach. Several studies have shown that if doctors at the referring site are involved with the consultation they learn from the experience and over time make fewer referrals.

Another approach is to task shift through continuing medical educa-tion of staff, both doctors and nurses, at the designated hospital. This would lead to better initial management and possibly fewer referrals. Tele-education using videoconferencing or recorded lectures is feasible in our setting. Another approach is to use videoconferencing to take advantage of the slightly better capacity in the private sector. International cross-border telemedicine taking advantage of psychiatrists in better-resourced HICs is feasible, but there are issues of language, culture, and legal and ethical concerns.

Political Will

The government has shown, in the National eHealth Strategy, its intention to harness information and communication technologies to facilitate implementation of the proposed National Health Insurance. One of the early outputs of the strategy was the development of a National Telemedicine Strategy. This was developed in 2012 but has still not been released. The provincial Departments of Health largely pay lip service to telemedicine, as they do not have the staff to manage it or funds to support it. Several do not mention it in their 5-year strategic plans. The recent adoption of MomConnect for registration of pregnancy by the National Department of Health shows some commitment and political will.

Infrastructure

Videoconference-based telemental health requires adequate bandwidth. The South African Guidelines for Telemental Health acknowledge the problem and require a minimum of 256 kb/s for videoconference consultation. Until recently, few hospitals had sufficient Internet protocol (IP) bandwidth to meet this standard and videoconferencing has required ISDN lines or more recently Asymmetric Digital Subscriber Line (ADSL) connections. As technology continues to advance, the need to have expensive dedicated videoconferencing units is beginning to fall away to be replaced with desktop videoconferencing. What is not always achievable is the ability to pan, tilt, and zoom the cameras. Cost still remains a major barrier to widespread videoconference-based telemental healthcare in the public sector.

Legal and Ethical Issues

The introduction of telemedicine services always raises legal and ethical issues. This is of particular importance when dealing with a vulnerable group. Concerns are mostly about licensure, liability, jurisdiction, quality of care, remuneration, and compliance with data privacy and security legislation or regulations. Ethical guidelines were developed for phase one of the National Telemedicine System in 1999. These were rudimentary, adapted from a code of conduct for commercial telemedicine equipment vendors and were largely irrelevant.[35] The Health Professions Council of South Africa (HPCSA) is a statutory body that licenses health professionals and develops ethical guidelines. They have been working on guidelines for the ethical practice of telemedicine in South Africa for over 8 years. In the absence of ethical guidelines, clinical, technical, and operational Guidelines for the Practice of Telemental Health in South Africa were developed before initiating a service. The guidelines were adapted from those of the American Telemedicine Association and take local infrastructure and circumstances into account.[28]

The draft guidelines of the HPCSA require written informed consent for telemedicine encounters, with copies held by the patient and the health professional consulted. Consent must cover all aspects of the telemedicine consultation including consent to use the appropriate and relevant technology, and details of data encryption and password protection. All electronic communications including practitioner authentication and the doctor's practice number must be stored and filed in the patient's medical file.

To be valid, consent must be fully understood and should ideally be obtained in the patient's first language. Indigenous languages have not kept pace with the growth of information and communication technologies. It has been shown that only 7% of isiZulu-speaking rural patients understood the meaning of the first sentence of the standard telemedicine consent, "I consent to a telemedicine consultation," that had been translated into isiZulu by five isiZulu first-language speakers, including a translator, a surgeon, and an IT consultant.[36]

The draft HPCSA guidelines also require a prior doctor–patient relationship and initial face-to-face consultation before a telemedicine consultation. This would limit telemental health to follow-up visits and runs contrary to the government's vision of telemedicine as a means of providing rural patients with access to specialists, and improving their quality of care.

Telemental health consultations to date have been viewed as a second-opinion service, with the referring doctor remaining responsible for the patient. This is in keeping with World Medical Association's guidelines.

CONCLUSION

There is little doubt that South Africa, like the rest of Africa, urgently needs better provision of mental health services. The problem is the shortage of psychiatrists and other health professionals working in mental health. Videoconference-based telemedicine adds extra steps to routine workflow, but saves psychiatrists from having to travel to rural hospitals. It also provides the opportunity for psychiatrists in the private sector to offer their services at rural sites. Tele-education for staff at designated district hospitals will improve their knowledge and raise awareness of videoconferencing for telemental health. With a National eHealth Strategy and Guidelines for the Practice of Telemental Health already published, the task is to scale up the fledgling service in KwaZulu-Natal and replicate it throughout the country. Pragmatic solutions are needed to resolve the problems posed in the HPCSA's draft Guidelines for the Practice of Telemedicine and Telemental Health in South Africa.

REFERENCES

1.   Mars M, Ramlall S, Kaliski S. Forensic telepsychiatry: a possible solution for South Africa? African Journal of Psychiatry. 2012;15(4):244–247.
2.   Wynchank S, Fortuin J. Telepsychiatry in South Africa: present and future. South African Journal of Psychiatry. 2010;1(1):16–19.

3. Health Systems Trust. Health indicators. http://www.hst.org.za/content/health-indicators. Published 2015. Accessed June 28, 2015.

4. World Bank. South Africa. http://data.worldbank.org/country/south-africa. Published 2015. Accessed June 28, 2015.

5. World Bank. Poverty and equity. World Bank, 2015. http://povertydata.worldbank.org/poverty/country/ZAF. Published 2015. Accessed June 28, 2015.

6. World Health Organization. Global Health Observatory data repository. http://apps.who.int/gho/data/node.country.country-ZAF. Published 2015. Accessed June 28, 2015.

7. Rotheram-Borus MJ, Richter L, van RH, et al. Project Masihambisane: a cluster randomised controlled trial with peer mentors to improve outcomes for pregnant mothers living with HIV. Trials. 2011;12:2.

8. Rochat TJ, Tomlinson M, Barnighausen T, Newell ML, Stein A. The prevalence and clinical presentation of antenatal depression in rural South Africa. Journal of Affective Disorders. 2011;135(1–3):362–373.

9. Hirschowitz R, Orkin M. Trauma and mental health in South Africa. Social Indicators Research. 1997;41(1):169–182.

10. Benatar SR. The challenges of health disparities in South Africa. South African Medical Journal. 2013;103(3):154–155.

11. World Health Organization. World health statistics 2015. Luxembourg: WHO; 2015.

12. Econex. Updated GP and specialist numbers for SA. Health Reform Note 7. http://www.econex.co.za. Published 2010. Accessed June 28, 2015.

13. South African Society of Psychiatrists. Psychiatric services. http://www.sasop.co.za/D_UC_PsychServices.asp. Published 2015. Accessed June 28, 2015.

14. van Wyk B-E, van Oudtshoorn B, Gericke N. Medicinal plants of South Africa. Pretoria: Briza Publications; 1997.

15. Sorsdahl K, Stein DJ, Flisher AJ. Traditional healer attitudes and beliefs regarding referral of the mentally ill to Western doctors in South Africa. Transcultural Psychiatry. 2010;47(4):591–609.

16. Ramlall S, Chipps J, Mars M. Impact of the South African Mental Health Care Act No. 17 of 2002 on regional and district hospitals designated for mental health care in KwaZulu-Natal. South African Medical Journal. 2010;100(10):667–670.

17. Department of Health Republic of South Africa. National Mental Health Policy Framework and Strategic Plan 2013–2020. Pretoria: Government Printer; 2013.

18. Burns J. Mental health services funding and development in KwaZulu-Natal: A tale of inequity and neglect. South African Medical Journal. 2010;100(10):662–666.

19. Department of Health Republic of South Africa. National eHealth Strategy South Africa 2012/13–2016/17. Pretoria: Government Press; 2012.

20. Mars M. Telemedicine in KwaZulu-Natal: from failure to cautious optimism. Journal of Telemedicine and Telecare. 2007;13(SUPPL. 3):57–59.

21. Naidoo S, Mars M. Telemedicine in the public sector in South Africa: an overview. Telemedicine and eHealth Updates. Knowledge Resources. 2015;8:381–385.

22. Jack C, Singh Y, Mars M. Pitfalls in computer housekeeping by doctors and nurses in KwaZulu-Natal: no malicious intent. BMC Medical Ethics. 2013;14Suppl 1: S8.

23. Wynchank S, Fortuin J. African telenursing: what is it and what's special about it? 2nd International Conference on eHealth, Telemedicine, and Social Medicine, eTELEMED 2010. St. Maarten. 2010; 17–22.

24. Ramlall S, Chipps J, Mars M. A survey on the impact of the South African Mental Health Care Act No. 17 of 2002 on designated hospitals in KwaZulu-Natal. South African Medical Journal. 2013;100(10):667–670.

25. Chipps J, Mars M. Readiness of health-care institutions in KwaZulu-Natal to implement telepsychiatry. Journal of Telemedicine and Telecare. 2012;18(3):133–137.

26. Chipps J, Ramlall S, Madigoe T, King H, Mars M. Developing telepsychiatry services in KwaZulu-Natal: an action research study. African Journal of Psychiatry. 2012;15(4):255–263.

27. Chipps J, Ramlall S, Mars M. A telepsychiatry model to support psychiatric outreach in the public sector in South Africa. African Journal of Psychiatry. 2012;15(4):264–270.

28. Chipps J, Ramlall S, Mars M. Practice guidelines for videoconference-based telepsychiatry in South Africa. African Journal of Psychiatry. 2012;15(4):271–282.

29. Chipps J, Ramlall S, Mars M. Videoconference-based education for psychiatry registrars at the University of KwaZulu-Natal, South Africa. African Journal of Psychiatry. 2012;15(4):248–254.

30. Rotheram-Borus MJ, Tomlinson M, le Roux IM, et al. A cluster randomised controlled effectiveness trial evaluating perinatal home visiting among South African mothers/infants. PLoS One. 2014;9(10):e105934.

31. Tsai AC, Tomlinson M, Dewing S, et al. Antenatal depression case finding by community health workers in South Africa: feasibility of a mobile phone application. Archives of Women's Mental Health. 2014;17(5):423–431.

32. Deglise C, Suggs LS, Odermatt P. Short message service (SMS) applications for disease prevention in developing countries. Journal of Medical Internet Research. 2012;14(1):e3.

33. South African Depression and Anxiety Group. Patients as partners. http://www.sadag.org/index.php?option=com_content&view=article&id=206:patients-as-partners&catid=61&Itemid=143. Published 2015. Accessed June 28, 2015.

34. MomConnect. Reducing maternal and child mortality through strengthening primary health care. http://www.rmchsa org/momconnect/. Published 2010. Accessed June 28, 2015.

35. Mars M, Jack C. Why is telemedicine a challenge to the regulators. South African Journal of Bioethics and Law. 2010;3(2):55–58.

36. Jack C, Singh Y, Hlombe B, Mars M. Language, cultural brokerage and informed consent: will technological terms impede telemedicine use? South African Journal of Bioethics and Law. 2014;7(1):14–18.

5

Telemental Health in
the Middle East

HUSSAM JEFEE-BAHLOUL AND ZAKARIA ZAYOUR

The Middle East (ME) is a unique region of the world with a rich history, culture, and tradition. Ongoing conflicts, however, continue to bring unrest and instability to that area, leaving negative consequences on economies, development, and healthcare. As in other parts of the world, mental health in the ME is one of the major public health concerns.

Globally, the estimated lifetime prevalence of common mental disorders including substance abuse is 29.2%, with one in every five adults (17.6%) having experienced a mental disorder within the past 12 months.[1] In the ME, only a few general population studies have been conducted to look at the prevalence of mental disorders. In Iraq, between 2007 and 2008, the estimated lifetime prevalence of any mental disorder according to the Iraqi Mental Health Survey (IMHS) ($n = 4,332$ adults) was reported to be 18.8%.[2] This cohort analysis showed significantly increasing lifetime prevalence of most disorders across generations, most pronounced for panic disorder and post-traumatic stress disorder. A comparable large-scale epidemiological study of adult mental disorders in Lebanon (n = 2,857 adults) showed a lifetime and 12-month prevalence estimates of any mental disorder of 25.8% and 17.0%, respectively.[3] These estimates place mental disorders among the most commonly occurring health problems in Lebanon.[4] Moreover, in Israel, a lifetime *Diagnostic and Statistical Manual* (DSM) diagnosis was found in 17.6% of respondents in the World Health Organization (WHO) World Mental Health Survey.[5]

Mental and substance use disorders are notable contributors to the global burden of disease (GBD), directly accounting for about 7.4% of disease burden worldwide.[6] This is especially noticeable in the ME region. For instance, depression is the third leading cause of disability-adjusted life years (DALYs) in the ME but is the 11th worldwide.[7] A systematic analysis for the Global Burden of Disease Study 2013 showed that in the ME, Major Depressive Disorder (MDD) was the leading cause of years lived with disability (YLDs) in Jordan, Syria, and Palestine and the second leading cause in Iran, Kuwait, Lebanon, Oman, Turkey, and the United Arab Emirates (UAE).[8] The GBD study in 2010 had already noted that armed conflict had increased the prevalence of MDD in Middle East/ North Africa region, which in turn led to a higher burden ranking.[7] In fact, research on the impact of war, violence, and political unrest on the prevalence of depression and PTSD has shown an association with higher levels of depression and PTSD.[9] A recent systematic review on the mental health of children and adolescents in areas of armed conflict in the Middle East estimated the prevalence of PTSD to be 5%–8% in Israel, 23%–70% in Palestine, and 10%–30% in Iraq.[10]

Despite the significant burden of mental illness, most of the countries in the ME lack mental health systems in terms of financial resources, manpower, infrastructure, and legislation, according to the data provided by Jacob et al.[11] (see chapter 1, table 1.1). The data show that Middle Eastern countries spend significantly less of their GDP on health compared with Western countries. Moreover, it shows that the number of psychiatrists per 100,000 people is five or less in all the countries in the ME except Israel, where it is 13.7. According to the WHO Mental Health Atlas

2011, there are only 0.27 outpatient facilities per 100,000 in the Eastern Mediterranean Region (EMR; includes the majority of the Middle Eastern countries) compared with 0.61 globally and 1.47 in Europe.

Given the scarcity of available mental health services and the substantial impact of mental illness, innovative approaches to help bridge the gap, including the use of technology, have been suggested. In the following sections, we review the state of telemedicine and telemental health (TMH) in the ME and analyze the barriers and suggest facilitators for implementation of TMH services in the region.

TELEMEDICINE IN THE MIDDLE EAST

Telemedicine in the Middle East is not yet as implemented or studied as it is in high-income countries. The telemedicine experience in the ME has varied considerably among the different individual countries due to multiple factors including finances, technology, infrastructure, culture, and others. The Kingdom of Saudi Arabia (KSA) and the UAE are among those countries that have recognized the importance of information and communications technology (ICT) and made considerable progress over the years in several ICT fields. For example, in KSA, the National Telemedicine Network comprises at least 20 connected hospitals that use remote operations as well as voice- and videoconferencing services.[12] The KSA also has the most advanced mobile health system in the region.[13] In 2014, the UAE, in partnership with a Swiss telemedicine provider, opened the Abu Dhabi Telemedicine Centre, the first center to provide 24/7 medical teleconsultation services in the country.

In Bahrain, six telemedical screening units in different parts of the country were used to screen 17,490 diabetic patients for diabetic retinopathy (DR); the study proved that a telemedicine-based screening program for DR was both feasible and effective in detecting DR.[14] In turn, Egypt has had a successful experience with using telepathology in a project launched in 2003 at Cairo University; this telemedical practice helped provide better medical care and reduce cost and time compared with the classic approach.[15] In Turkey, telemedicine was used in decision-making and follow-up of burn patients and was found to be successful and cost-effective; it decreased mortality and the need to transfer patients to the major referral burn center.[16]

TELEMENTAL HEALTH IN THE MIDDLE EAST

A literature search of four engines (Pubmed, Ovid, Google Scholar, and IMEMR) for publications that reported or addressed TMH in the ME was done.[17] Case reports, systematic reviews, opinion articles, and clinical trials were searched. Eleven ($n = 11$) publications were found (all publications in English, except one Farsi paper[18]). An updated search revealed one additional publication along with one report in press (Table 5.1). These reports tackled different aspects of the TMH systems in the ME such as the online patient–physician relationship, attitudes toward TMH, and feasibility and challenges of implementation of TMH.

The online therapeutic work alliance was studied in a randomized controlled trial that used an Internet-based, culturally adapted cognitive-behavioral therapy (CBT) technique on Iraqis suffering from post-traumatic stress disorder (PTSD).[19] The intervention is an Internet-based "interapy" (Internet + therapy) CBT approach adapted from a Dutch CBT-based intervention and uses asynchronous, text-based communication between the therapist and the patient. The treatment involved giving participants semiweekly 45-minute CBT-based writing assignments over a 5-week period (10 essays in total). In turn, eight therapists provide feedback and written instructions for the following assignment. The therapists are native Arabic-speaking psychologists or psychiatrists who live in Iraq, Palestine, Syria, the Emirates, or Europe. The primary outcome measure of this randomized controlled trial, which involved ($n = 55$) Iraqi patients with PTSD, was the Working Alliance Inventory (WAI) administered at midtreatment (session 4) and post-treatment (sessions 10). The authors also collected Posttraumatic Diagnostic Scale (PDS) scores at baseline and post-treatment. The study showed that a positive and therapeutic online

TABLE 5.1 PUBLISHED STUDIES OF TELEMENTAL HEALTH IN THE MIDDLE EAST

	Country	Mode of Telemental Health	N	RCT	Study Description	Clinical Outcome	Findings
Jefee-Bahloul (2015)[22]	Syria	Store & Feed	30	N/A	Attitudes toward TMH	Perception of effectiveness of S&F, willingness to make referrals through S&F, barriers	HCPs are open to implementing S&F and believe it is helpful while acknowledging cultural, financial, and technical barriers
Jefee-Bahloul (2015)[47]	Syria	Store & Forward	N/A	N/A	Implementation of S&F TMH network to provide consultations and clinical supervision	N/A	Using S&F was helpful but there was concern about the scope of the advice given. S&F can be potentially used for global academic teaching as well
Wagner (2012)[23]	Iraq	Internet-based, Asynchronous	15	N/A	"Interapy"; asynchronous writing assignments and interactions between patients with PTSD and therapists.	PDS, HSCL-25, Quality of Life	Significant improvement of clinical outcomes

(continued)

TABLE 5.1 CONTINUED

	Country	Mode of Telemental Health	N	RCT	Study Description	Clinical Outcome	Findings
Wagner (2012)[19]	Iraq	Internet-based, Asynchronous	55	Y	CBT	WAI, PDS	Positive online relationship, symptom improvement
Werner (2004)[21]	Israel	N/A	1,204	N/A	Theoretical attitudes assessment toward telemental health	N/A	Moderate willingness to use telemental health
Modai (2006)[45]	Israel	Videoconferencing	66	Y-CT	Videoconferencing vs. face-to-face psychiatric treatments.	cost analysis, treatment adherence, clinical safety (BPRS, CGI), patients' and therapists' satisfaction	More adherence in VC group, similar satisfaction between the groups, VC group had higher costs compared to face-to-face.
Aviv (2006)[24]	Israel	Telephone based	12	N/A	Treatment of adolescents who have school refusal with telehypnosis.	School attendance	Improved school attendance in the majority of participants.

Study	Country	Platform	N		Intervention	Measures	Results
Ozkan (2013)[25]	Turkey	Telephone based	62	Y	Family intervention; psychoeducation inpatient followed by telepsychiatric follow-up (via telephone) after discharge.	The Level of Expressed Emotion Scale, Zarit Family Burden scale, and Beck Depression scale.	Significant improvement on all scales in intervention group compared with control.
Mazhari (2012)[18]	Iran	N/A	N/A	N/A	Description of the challenges facing tele-mental health implementation in Iran	N/A	Telemental health is not implemented in Iran. Some of the barriers are financial, technical, and concerns about confidentiality
Deldar (2011)[27]	Iran	Internet based	420	N/A	Content Evaluation of ask-a-doctor website.	N/A	The most frequent questions were of mental health and women's health.

(continued)

TABLE 5.1 CONTINUED

	Country	Mode of Telemental Health	N	RCT	Study Description	Clinical Outcome	Findings
Jefee-Bahloul (2014)[48]	Jordan (Syrian refugees)	Videoconferencing	N/A	N/A	Videoconferencing-based telemental health supervision of mental health treatments in a conflict setting.	N/A	Telemental health can be useful for supervision, and consultations to mental health providers in conflict areas.
Jefee-Bahloul (2014)[20]	Turkey (Syrian refugees)	N/A	354	N/A	Theoretical attitudes toward telemental health in a sample of Syrian refugees in Turkey	HADStress	Despite prevalence of psychological stress there is a partial hesitance toward telemental health in this sample.
Quackenbush (2012)[28]	Middle East	Internet-based, Virtual Reality	1	N/A	Psychotherapy provided in the "second life" virtual environment by text messaging between two avatars (client and therapist).	N/A	Demonstration of feasibility of virtual therapy.

N = Number of participants in the study if applicable, RCT = Randomized controlled trial, N/A: Not applicable, CT = Controlled trial but not randomized.

relationship can be established and maintained as evidenced by high ratings on the WAI composite scores. The study also confirmed the findings of the previous study that "interapy" is effective in decreasing PTSD symptoms.

Three other reports addressed the attitudes of both patients and providers toward using TMH services. In one study, a sample (n = 354) of Syrian refugees in a primary care clinic in Kilis, Turkey, were surveyed. The participants answered the HADStress screening tool and were asked about their openness to referral to mental health and TMH services. Of the surveyed sample, 41.8% had scores on HADStress that correlate to PTSD. However, only 34% of the whole sample reported a perceived need to see a psychiatrist, and of those only 45% were open to TMH, indicating "partial acceptance" to TMH in this sample. Some of the reasons for not accepting TMH included "security of the Internet," "better communication in person," "not knowing what is telepsychiatry."[20] Other aspects of this study are discussed later in this chapter.

Another study from Israel assessed the attitudes toward using telemedicine for psychiatric care.[21] Phone interviews of (n = 1,420) patients were conducted to measure the "willingness" to use TMH, defined as subjective perception about using these services in a hypothetical situation in which they feel anxious, sad, or distressed. The authors concluded that participants had a relatively high willingness to use TMH, with a mean score of 3.2 on a 5-point Likert scale (with 1 showing least willingness and 5 showing most willingness). Participants' willingness was found to be affected by their attitudes toward telemedicine, their attitudes toward the patient–physician relationship, and the level of technology anxiety.

A more recent study on TMH in Syria used electronic surveys to assess the attitudes of Syrian nonpsychiatric healthcare providers (HCPs) toward using a store-and-forward (S&F) system to receive mental health consultation.[22] Even though the majority of the respondents had little or no prior experience with TMH, they were open to such services, and 77% believed that patients would benefit from S&F consultations. On the other hand, they did acknowledge that cultural (68%), financial (84%), and technical (80%) considerations are barriers to implementing such services. The report also highlighted the feasibility of conducting electronic surveys of healthcare workers in a humanitarian setting.

Five reports looked at the use of different TMH services: "interapy" (therapy over the Internet), telehypnosis, telephonic psychoeducation, teleconsultation to patients, teleconsultation and supervision to HCPs, and "virtual therapy."

In an efficacy noncontrolled study in Iraq, Wagner used "interapy," explained earlier, with ($n = 15$) Iraqi participants with PTSD.[23] Three scales, administered pre- and post-intervention, were used: the PDS, which rates the severity of PTSD symptoms; the Hopkins Symptoms Checklist-25 (HSCL-25), which evaluates symptoms of anxiety and depression; and the EUROHIS-QOL eight-item scale, which measures four domains of quality of life (psychological, physical, social, and environmental). Significant treatment benefits were observed for all the evaluated domains (reduction in PTSD, depression, and anxiety symptoms as well as improvement in quality of life) thus demonstrating the efficacy of "interapy." Furthermore, the authors argued that the anonymity of this Internet-based program offers an opportunity to overcome the hesitance in seeking mental health treatment given the stigmatization and shame that accompanies mental illness in Iraq and neighboring countries.

Another modality of TMH was studied in Israel and aimed at treating adolescent school refusal.[24] Hypnosis conducted over the phone, or "telehypnosis," was provided to ($n = 12$) adolescents who had already failed various psychopharmacological and psychotherapeutic interventions and had a combined average of 65 weeks of absence. The participants were asked to contact their therapists using their cellular phones whenever their anxiety level reached 5 out of 10 using a 10-point anxiety scale (1 = no anxiety, 10 = high anxiety), whether they were still at home, on their way to school, or even after they arrived at school. Follow-up results in 1 year showed that eight students were able to retain full attendance, three showed partial improvement in their attendance, and only one failed to improve and eventually went back to avoiding school.

A Turkish study looked at the use of TMH to provide follow-up on psychoeducation provided to primary caregivers of patients with schizophrenia.[25] Psychoeducation has been shown in previous studies to decrease caregiver psychological burden.[26] In this randomized controlled trial, the experimental group of caregivers received face-to-face (F2F) psychoeducation during hospitalization followed by telephonic follow-up sessions ($n = 32$) while the control group did not receive either intervention during the study period ($n = 30$). At the end of the study, mean scores of all three outcome measures—Level of Expressed Emotion Scale (LEE), Beck Depression Inventory (BDI), and the Zarit Family Burden Assessment Scale—were significantly decreased in the intervention arm (F2F + TMH) compared with controls. Because the control group did not receive F2F psychoeducation, it is not possible to look at the direct effect of the telephonic sessions (i.e., TMH) on the treatment group; however, it can be implied from this study that TMH can be used as part of a psychoeducation program for caregivers.

A report from Iran looked at the use of teleconsultation using an "ask-the-doctor" service, where participants send private enquiries to physicians using a textual asynchronous Internet-based model.[27] Questions related to mental health were among the most frequently asked questions, and the authors argued that the online consultation can be used to overcome patients' cultural reluctance to discuss such sensitive topics. No clinical outcome measure was reported in the paper.

Providing mental health consultations and supervision to HCPs using a store-and-forward (S&F) system was described in a Syrian pilot study in 2014.[22] The Syrian Telemental Health Network (STMH), a global TMH system, provided these services to HCPs at different Syrian refugee clinics in Turkey, Jordan, Lebanon, and Syria. The authors describe how the S&F technology, which uses asynchronous (nonlive) communication, can be a viable alternative to videoconferencing especially in humanitarian conflict settings or unstable low- to middle-income countries where that latter technology has its limitations.

Finally, one study reported the use the "second-life" online game to provide "virtual reality psychotherapy" to a patient in the ME. The therapist, located in the United States did not have a videoconferencing encounter with patient; rather, interaction was solely through text exchange between two "avatars" in a virtual environment and was reported to have been a feasible and beneficial approach despite the raised ethical and therapeutic concerns.[28]

Cost, barriers, and feasibility of implementing TMH systems in the ME were discussed in the three remaining reports. In Israel/Palestinian territories, Modai et al. reported a cost-effectiveness controlled study to compare mental healthcare services administered via videoconferencing versus traditional F2F interviewing.[29] Data was collected from a group of ($n = 39$) patients who agreed to receive care via TMH videoconferencing and a control group of ($n = 42$) matched patients who continued receiving F2F services. This data was also compared with that of the previous year. The clinical outcome measures used were Brief Psychiatric Rating Scale (BPRS), Clinical Global Impression Scale (CGI), Patient and Therapist Satisfaction Questionnaires (PSQ and TSQ), and a financial cost analysis. Even though CGI scores remained stable, BPRS scores were significantly decreased, indicating improvement in symptoms in both groups. Moreover, both patients and therapists expressed satisfaction with TMH. However, the cost analysis showed that an hour-long videoconferencing session was 32% more expensive that its F2F counterpart. This value decreased to 10.6% when the travel expenses of TMH patients during the preceding year were included in the analysis. The authors argued that this data cannot be generalized due to the limited sample size. More about the financial barriers to adopting TMH in the ME is discussed later in this chapter.

Another report from Iran (in Farsi) looked at the barriers facing the implementation of a TMH system there, and identified several obstacles including privacy and physician compensation.[18] No TMH services were described in the paper, but the authors discussed the potential establishment of such a system once more information on instituting TMH systems in this part of the world becomes available.

The third report was a case example of feasibility of TMH supervision in the humanitarian setting. The report describes conducting videoconferencing-based supervision (from the United States to Jordan) of a psychiatrist in Jordan who is involved in treating Syrian refugees. The report highlights multiple challenges to such videoconferencing-based telesupervision. The Internet connection was of modest quality, which resulted in poor-quality videoconferencing. Also, the treating psychiatrist was not available on every occasion. This is due to the time demands, the nature of work in such humanitarian settings, and the lack of remuneration for this collaborative telesupervision work.[30]

BARRIERS TO IMPLEMENTATION OF TELEMENTAL HEALTH IN THE MIDDLE EAST

This section discusses barriers for implementation of telemental health in the ME and provide assessment and recommendations based on a synthesized review of the published studies and on the author's personal experience. Four main barriers to implementing TMH in the ME are frequently observed: cultural, technical, financial, and regulatory.

Cultural Barriers

The culture in the ME entails a great emphasis on close social interactions and interpersonal relationships, and such societies expect direct doctor–patient communication.[31] Using technology in providing medical services in this context is expected to face several barriers. Moreover, the unfamiliarity with technology in certain cultures is another major hurdle that could thwart the adoption of TMH services. It has been shown that lack of knowledge of technology, especially among elderly patients, increases reluctance to use TMH services.[31,32] This is in contrast to younger, educated patients, who exhibit great comfort with such services.[33,34,35] both patients and providers show these attitudes and reluctance.

Patients in the ME often express concerns about physicians' culture (tradition and religion), the technology being used, security, and privacy and confidentiality.[36] In the PASSPORT study discussed earlier in this chapter, in which Syrian refugees were surveyed on their openness to psychiatry and telepsychiatry, privacy, distortions to the doctor–patient relationship, and unfamiliarity with the technology were reasons behind the hesitance to use TMH.[20]

Other cultural factors that might have an impact on the application of TMH in the ME are age, gender, and religion. As mentioned earlier, several studies have shown that younger patients are more comfortable and more open to TMH compared with the older population.[21,31,33] In the ME, females are less satisfied with mental healthcare services than men.[37] This could be due to the fact that females in the ME are generally more conservative and have less public exposure than men.[37] In the PASSPORT study, females were less likely to accept TMH ($p = .64$) compared with males and were more likely to accept F2F psychiatry ($p < .05$).

Even though the PASSPORT study did not include religion as a variable, most of the surveyed participants were actually from the northern—more conservative—part of Syria. The impact of religion on the perception and attitude toward TMH was taken into account in one of the Israeli studies mentioned earlier. The study showed that religious patients were less willing to use TMH compared with secular patients.[21]

Provider-related barriers to TMH are lack of knowledge and technical expertise as well as the need for training (e.g., use of technology, verbal and nonverbal communication through technology).[36] The value of physical interaction is also a commonly noted reason for reluctance among providers.[36] Moreover, time constraints and remuneration issues can add to the providers' hesitance toward the use of technology.[36] In conclusion, cultural concerns bring about significant obstacles to implementing an effective TMH system in the ME. Approaches to overcome these cultural barriers include training providers and increasing their knowledge of the technology as well as promoting awareness of its feasibility. In turn, patients' acceptance can be enhanced through programs designed to increase public awareness of the technology and of the value of TMH. For example, in a Swedish study that involved providing TMH services (videoconferencing) to Middle Eastern patients residing in Sweden and Denmark, the participants reported a high level of satisfaction and willingness to use TMH;[38]

the results suggest that cultural acceptance of TMH is possible with more experience with this technology.

Infrastructural and Technical Barriers

Some countries in the ME possess the infrastructure required for the implementation of telemedicine (e.g., Israel, Turkey, Jordan, UAE) but many others unfortunately do not (e.g., Syria, Iraq, Iran). Two fundamental elements for establishing a telemedicine/TMH network are electricity and Internet. However, electricity is not available 24/7 in some Middle Eastern countries like Lebanon (of note is that mobile technology can be used to overcome the unreliability of electricity[39]). Access to high network bandwidth capacity is also challenging to obtain; high bandwidth capacity ensures better resolution and sound, two elements that are vital to the therapeutic relationship.[40] Another obstacle, mostly in remote settings, is the shortage of trained technical support staff who can handle technical difficulties or problems as well as medical personnel available for emergencies.

To overcome these barriers, more pilot studies are needed in order to better advocate for telemedicine and encourage the local governments to invest in this field. In investigating the readiness of ME countries for implementing telemedicine, Alajlani[36] developed a framework that can be applied in the preimplementation phase. The authors surveyed and interviewed stakeholders (physicians, patients, technicians, engineers, and decision makers) in both Syria and Jordan in 2010 (prior to the Syrian Civil War). The recommendations, provided to organizations and agencies interested in creating telemedicine systems in the ME, included partnering with local public and private as well as international organizations, ensuring availability of technical infrastructure and human resources, intensive training of healthcare personnel, and staying up to date with the country's policies (Box. 5.1).[36,41] Even though the guideline framework was formulated based on work in only Syria and Jordan, the authors argued that it can be generalized and applied to other countries in the ME.

Box 5.1   GUIDELINE FRAMEWORK FOR IMPLEMENTATION OF TELEMEDICINE PROJECTS IN THE MIDDLE EAST

Fully understand the readiness of telemedicine in the country.

Study the needs of the country and its requirement for telemedicine applications, because the needs for adopting telemedicine in one country can be different from the needs of other countries.

Study the country policies and be sure that the law and the regulations support your project.

Understand all current government policies regarding telecommunication and healthcare service provision, as governments may apply new rules and tax regarding telecommunication.

Check the policies regularly and always keep yourself updated, as there are always new regulations regarding telecommunication.

Check the customs policies in order to know what devices you are allowed to import and what you are not allowed to import. Ensure that the infrastructure is prepared and robust.

Consider the status of the infrastructure and the limitations of telecommunications in the country because there might be restrictions on telecommunication between your country and other countries.

Study the availability of essential resources, both technical and human.

Provide intensive training to healthcare staff through seminars, courses, and online conferences, and facilitate all the training resources (books, journals, computers, etc.) to keep the staff updated and motivated about the application of telemedicine.

Apply an efficient model to facilitate payment transactions and consider that the modern methods of payment such as credit cards and e-banking are newly introduced in some countries (e.g., Syria).

Differentiate between urban and rural requirements, as there can be large differences between the two areas in some countries (e.g., Jordan).

Create a partnership with government organizations (public–private partnership) to gain their support and ensure smooth progress of the telemedicine application.

Convince decision makers of the viability of the project before the project.

Establish a connection with international health organizations (e.g., WHO) to gain support and help.

Promote the project properly through campaigns and publicity so it gains acceptance by everyone.

Employ local resources in the development of the telemedicine application so that people will be motivated and more involved in the application.

Conduct feasibility studies and cost-effectiveness analysis with consideration of any policy restrictions, such as online banking.

Understand the social and cultural requirements (religion, language, etc.), since people in the Middle East hold on to traditions.

Consider the relationship between your country and other countries that may be connected via telemedicine, as there may be some specific issues regarding communication and medical relevant to a particular country and consider that some countries (e.g., Syria) has restriction on technology as it is still under sanction from the United States.

Source: Adapted from Alajlani M. Issues facing the application of telemedicine in developing countries: Hashemite Kingdom of Jordan and Syrian Arab Republic. School of Information Systems, Computing and Mathematics. 2010.

Legal and Ethical Barriers

Different views of the role of the healthcare system shape the legal system, which leads to variation in health-related legal frameworks among countries.[42] As telemedicine has not yet been established as a common medical practice in the ME, there are no regulations or bylaws that control it. Once implemented, issues such as medicolegal concerns, licensing requirements, and regulation and quality assurance are likely to emerge. These concerns, especially those related to patient confidentiality, can affect patient's acceptance of TMH[43] and thus call for the need to develop policies and statutes to guarantee the safety of electronically transmitted information. Informed consent and the ability of patients to access their medical records are two considerations that should be thought of when putting together TMH systems.[44]

In order to establish an effective TMH system in the ME, effort should be made to develop the medicolegal system and ensure the presence of proper regulations and policies that control the practice of telemedicine and TMH. Without such a system, issues such as confidentiality, informed consent, and liability would be jeopardized, thus dramatically risking any chance of practicing telemedicine in the ME.

Financial Barriers

Funding TMH programs might not be a barrier in some Middle Eastern countries such as Qatar, Kuwait, and UAE, but it is a significant hurdle in other parts of the ME such as Jordan and Syria.[36] Alajlani speculates that the private sector is more likely to take the initiative in establishing telemedicine projects and adopt the technology given the little interest and support from the public sector.[36] While it has been shown that TMH is cost-effective in the developed world,[45] this is yet to be the case in the ME. In the Israeli randomized controlled trial discussed earlier, the cost analysis showed that services provided via videoconferencing were more expensive than those provided F2F (cost of hospitalization was 223% higher, and cost of sessions was 32% higher for TMH).[29] Therefore, attracting investors and stakeholders to this field will remain a challenge unless more studies demonstrate the cost-effectiveness in the ME. A reasonable first step would be to start with the less expensive S&F technology; nevertheless, this also needs to be confirmed by cost-effectiveness studies.

It is important to conceptualize these barriers as an amalgam of related reenforcing issues specific to each country in the region; they are entwined and interacting entities rather than isolated matters that can be addressed independently. For example, it is the combination of financial concerns and poor infrastructure that further contributes to the provider-related cultural reluctance to use telemedicine. In the absence of a proper electronic fee exchange system and governmental support services, active physician participation is unlikely to occur even if the appropriate TMH training and education were provided. Patients' cultural reluctance is significantly impacted by their countries' legal system, given the possibility of corruption and power abuse in some parts of the ME. Creating and enforcing appropriate protective laws and policies is needed in order to increase patients' comfort with using TMH services. Tackling these entwined sets of barriers necessitates a reconstructive process involving public and private sector, policymakers, and agencies of interest.

CONCLUSION

Given the available reports, the use of TMH services has not been feasible on a large scale in the ME yet. This is in part explained by the unreliable quality of telecommunication, the absence of clear medicolegal guidelines and regulations for TMH, and patients' and providers' reluctance to use this technology.[21,36,43,46] Despite these barriers, there are continuing efforts and experiences with TMH in the ME such as the Syrian Telemental Health Network alluded to earlier.

In summary, this chapter has focused on reviewing existing reports concerning implementation of TMH in the Middle East. Telemental health programs can be used to bridge a considerable mental health gap in the ME. It can facilitate access to quality mental health services for patients and serve as a training and educational tool to advance mental health workers' expertise. However, several barriers stand in the way of its implementation. Some countries in the ME enjoy stability, while several others are in a state of conflict. Different Middle Eastern countries have different perceptions and readiness levels toward using and establishing TMH systems. Evaluation of each country's unique cultural, financial, legal, and infrastructural conditions should guide the strategies for developing these systems.

REFERENCES

1. Steel Z, Marnane C, Iranpour C, et al. The global prevalence of common mental disorders: a systematic review and meta-analysis 1980–2013. International Journal of Epidemiology. 2014;43(2):476–493.

2. Alhasnawi S, Sadik S, Rasheed M, et al. The prevalence and correlates of DSM-IV disorders in the Iraq Mental Health Survey (IMHS). World Psychiatry. 2009;8(2):97–109.

3. Karam EG, Mneimneh ZN, Dimassi H, et al. Lifetime prevalence of mental disorders in Lebanon: first onset, treatment, and exposure to war. PLoS medicine. 2008;5(4):e61.

4. Karam EG, Mneimneh ZN, Karam AN, et al. Prevalence and treatment of mental disorders in Lebanon: a national epidemiological survey. Lancet. 2006;367(9515):1000–1006.

5. Kessler RC, Aguilar-Gaxiola S, Alonso J, et al. The global burden of mental disorders: an update from the WHO World Mental Health (WMH) surveys. Epidemiol Psichiatr Soc. 2009;18(1):23–33.

6. Whiteford HA, Degenhardt L, Rehm J, et al. Global burden of disease attributable to mental and substance use disorders: findings from the Global Burden of Disease Study 2010. Lancet. 2013;382(9904):1575–1586.

7. Ferrari AJ, Charlson FJ, Norman RE, et al. Burden of depressive disorders by country, sex, age, and year: findings from the Global Burden of Disease Study 2010. PLoS Medicine. 2013;10(11):e1001547.

8. Vos T, Barber RM, Bell B, et al. Global, regional, and national incidence, prevalence, and years lived with disability for 301 acute and chronic diseases and injuries in 188 countries, 1990–2013: a systematic analysis for the Global Burden of Disease Study 2013. Lancet. 386(9995):743–800.

9. Steel Z, Chey T, Silove D, Marnane C, Bryant RA, van Ommeren M. Association of torture and other potentially traumatic events with mental health outcomes among populations exposed to mass conflict and displacement: A systematic review and meta-analysis. JAMA. 2009;302(5):537–549.

10. Dimitry L. A systematic review on the mental health of children and adolescents in areas of armed conflict in the Middle East. Child: Care, Health and Development. 2012;38(2):153–161.

11. Jacob K, Sharan P, Mirza I, et al. Mental health systems in countries: where are we now? Lancet. 2007;370(9592):1061–1077.

12. Jaber MM, Ghani MKA, Herman NS. A review of adoption of telemedicine in Middle East countries: toward building Iraqi telemedicine framework. International Symposium on Research in Innovation and Sustainability 2014 (ISoRIS '14) 15-16 October 2014, Malacca, Malaysia.

13. Ababtain AF, Almulhim DA, Househ MS. The state of mobile health in the developing world and the Middle East. Paper presented at: ICIMTH2013.

14. Al Alawi E, Ahmed AA. Screening for diabetic retinopathy: the first telemedicine approach in a primary care setting in Bahrain. Middle East African Journal of Ophthalmology. 2012;19(3):295–298.

15. Ayad E. Virtual telepathology in Egypt, applications of WSI in Cairo University. Diagnostic Pathology. 2011;6(Suppl 1):S1. https://www.ncbi.nlm.nih.gov/pmc/articles/PMC3073202/pdf/1746-1596-6-S1-S1.pdf

16. Turk E, Karagulle E, Aydogan C, et al. Use of telemedicine and telephone consultation in decision-making and follow-up of burn patients: initial experience from two burn units. Burns. 37(3):415–419.

17. Jefee-Bahloul H. Telemental health in the Middle East: overcoming the barriers. Frontiers in Public Health. 2014;2:86.

18. Mazhari S, Bahaedin Beigi K. Telepsychiatry and its application in Iran. Iranian Journal of Psychiatry and Clinical Psychology. 2012;17(4):336–338.

19. Wagner B, Brand J, Schulz W, Knaevelsrud C. Online working alliance predicts treatment outcome for posttraumatic stress symptoms in Arab war-traumatized patients. Depression and Anxiety. 2012;29(7):646–651.

20. Jefee-Bahloul H, Moustafa MK, Shebl FM, Barkil-Oteo A. Pilot assessment and survey of Syrian refugees' psychological stress and openness to referral for telepsychiatry (PASSPORT Study). Telemedicine Journal and e-Health. 2014;20(10):977–979.

21. Werner P. Willingness to use telemedicine for psychiatric care. Telemedicine Journal and e-Health. 2004;10(3):286–293.

22. Jefee-Bahloul H, Duchen D, Barkil-Oteo A. Attitudes towards implementation of store-and-forward telemental health in humanitarian settings: survey of Syrian healthcare providers. Telemedicine Journal and e-Health 2015;22(1):31–35.

23. Wagner B, Schulz W, Knaevelsrud C. Efficacy of an Internet-based intervention for posttraumatic stress disorder in Iraq: a pilot study. Psychiatry Research. 2012;195(1–2):85–88.

24. Aviv A. Tele-hypnosis in the treatment of adolescent school refusal. American Journal of Clinical Hypnosis. 2006;49(1):31–40.

25. Ozkan B, Erdem E, Ozsoy SD, Zararsiz G. Effect of psychoeducation and telepsychiatric follow up given to the caregiver of the schizophrenic patient on family burden, depression and expression of emotion. Pakistan Journal of Medical Sciences. 2013;29(5):1122.

26. McWilliams S, Hill S, Mannion N, Fetherston A, Kinsella A, O'Callaghan E. Schizophrenia: a five-year follow-up of patient outcome following psychoeducation for caregivers. European Psychiatry. 2012;27(1):56–61.

27. Deldar K, Marouzi P, Assadi R. Teleconsultation via the web: an analysis of the type of questions that Iranian patients ask. Journal of Telemedicine and Telecare. 2011;17(6):324–327.

28. Quackenbush DM, Krasner A. Avatar therapy: where technology, symbols, culture, and connection collide. Journal of Psychiatric Practice. 2012;18(6):451–459.

29. Modai I, Jabarin M, Kurs R, Barak P, Hanan I, Kitain L. Cost effectiveness, safety, and satisfaction with video telepsychiatry versus face-to-face care in ambulatory settings. Telemedicine Journal and e-Health. 2006;12(5):515–520.

30. Jefee-Bahloul H. Use of telepsychiatry in areas of conflict: the Syrian refugee crisis as an example. Journal of Telemedicine and Telecare. 2014;20(3):165–166.

31. Nieves JE, Stack KM. Hispanics and telepsychiatry. Psychiatric Services. 2007;58(6):877–878; author reply 878.

32. Rohland BM, Saleh SS, Rohrer JE, Romitti PA. Acceptability of telepsychiatry to a rural population. Psychiatric Services. 2000;51(5):672–674.

33. Shore JH, Savin DM, Novins D, Manson SM. Cultural aspects of telepsychiatry. Journal of Telemedicine and Telecare. 2006;12(3):116–121.

34. Whitten P, Love B. Patient and provider satisfaction with the use of telemedicine: overview and rationale for cautious enthusiasm. Journal of Postgraduate Medicine. 2005;51(4).
35. Whitten PS, Mackert MS. Addressing telehealth's foremost barrier: provider as initial gatekeeper. International Journal of Technology Assessment in Health Care. 2005;21(4):517–521.
36. Alajlani M. Issues facing the application of telemedicine in developing countries: Hashemite Kingdom of Jordan and Syrian Arab Republic. School of Information Systems, Computing and Mathematics. 2010. http://ethos.bl.uk/OrderDetails.do?uin=uk.bl.ethos.534475
37. Bener A, Ghuloum S. Gender difference on patients' satisfaction and expectation towards mental health care. Nigerian Journal of Clinical Practice. 2013;16(3):285–291.
38. Mucic D. Transcultural telepsychiatry and its impact on patient satisfaction. Journal of Telemedicine and Telecare. 2010;16(5):237–242.
39. Alvarez-Jimenez M, Alcazar-Corcoles MA, Gonzalez-Blanch C, Bendall S, McGorry PD, Gleeson JF. Online, social media and mobile technologies for psychosis treatment: a systematic review on novel user-led interventions. Schizophrenia Research. 2014;156(1):96–106.
40. van Wynsberghe A, Gastmans C. Telepsychiatry and the meaning of in-person contact: a preliminary ethical appraisal. Medicine, Health Care and Philosophy. 2009;12(4):469–476.
41. Alajlani M, Clarke M. Effect of culture on acceptance of telemedicine in Middle Eastern countries: case study of Jordan and Syria. Telemedicine Journal and e-Health. 2013;19(4):305–311.
42. Kluge E-HW. Ethical and legal challenges for health telematics in a global world: telehealth and the technological imperative. International Journal of Medical Informatics. 2011;80(2):e1–e5.
43. Jefee-Bahloul H, Moustafa M, Shebl FM, Barkil-Oteo A. Pilot assessment and survey of Syrian refugees' psychological stress and openness to referral for telepsychiatry (PASSPORT study). Journal of Telemedicine and e-Health. 2014;20(10):977–979.
44. Kluge EH. Ethical and legal challenges for health telematics in a global world: telehealth and the technological imperative. International Journal of Medical Informatics. 2011;80(2):e1–e5.
45. Hyler SE, Gangure DP. A review of the costs of telepsychiatry. Psychiatric Services. 2003;54(7):976–980.
46. Alajlani M, Clarke M. Effect of culture on acceptance of telemedicine in Middle Eastern countries: case study of Jordan and Syria. Telemedicine and e-Health. 2013;19(4):305–311.
47. Jefee-Bahloul H, Barkil-Oteo A, Shukair N, Alraas W, Mahasneh W. Using a store-and-forward system to provide global telemental health supervision and training: a case from Syria. Academic Psychiatry. 2016;40(4):707–709.
48. Jefee-Bahloul H. Use of telepsychiatry in areas of conflict: the Syrian refugee crisis as an example. Journal of Telemedicine and Telecare. 2014;20(3):167–168.

6

Telemental Health in India

RANGASWAMY THARA, SUJIT JOHN, AND KOTTESWARA RAO

India, with a population of over 1.2 billion people, has less than 3,700 psychiatrists—that is, less than 0.05 per 10,000 population[1]—to provide mental health services. With an estimated 20% of the adult population in the country affected with a psychiatric disorder,[2] India faces a huge challenge in closing the treatment gap especially in rural areas, which have very few practicing mental health professionals.

The Indian government has tried to address this challenge by launching programs under the National Mental Health Program and the District Mental Health Program, which mandate that every district hospital in India have a psychiatrist. Implementation of this mandate is unfortunately hampered by the severe lack of available qualified professionals.

Under these circumstances, the use of telemedicine technology to provide psychiatric services offers a unique opportunity to reach out to the vast rural masses of India who would otherwise have no access to affordable mental healthcare service providers. The argument in favor of telepsychiatry is strengthening, with several studies showing that the accuracy of diagnosis and the levels of satisfaction in face-to-face consultations compared with consultations through telepsychiatry are similar.[3]

In theory, it is easier to set up a state-of-the-art telecommunication infrastructure in rural India, and thereby increase the reach of the limited number of urban specialists, than to make specialists available in places without them.[4] India's first telemedicine program was a pilot in 1998 that used the low-bandwidth, Integrated Services Digital Network (ISDN) technology for connectivity and networking,[5] and the first satellite-based telemedicine service was started in 2001.[6] There has since been a rapid growth of these services in India, facilitated by the growth of the information and communication industry in India. Paralleling this has been the growth of the e-health industry in India. It has also in part been fostered by the lack of any regulatory mechanism in place or any specific law dealing with the delivery of service through telemedicine.

At present this technology and service are ostensibly covered by the Indian Information Technology (Amendment) Act of 2008 and by laws on the practice of medicine such as the Medical Council of India Act of 1956 and the Code of Ethics Regulations of 2002. Processes are underway to develop a telemedicine act that would fall under the Ministry of Health and Family Welfare, Government of India. As a first step, a set of nonbinding guidelines, the *Recommended Guidelines & Standards for Practice of Telemedicine in India* was released in 2003. This document covered definitions and concepts; standards required for hardware, software, and clinical devices, including the security aspects; and the telemedicine process.

The initial focus and governmental support for telemedicine were in the fields of radiology, cardiology, and pathology,[7] followed by other specializations such as neurology, ophthalmology, and diabetes, all heavily dependent on image-based diagnosis.

While anecdotal references to telepsychiatry services in India are available, published data is sparse. Malhotra and colleagues[8] have reported the development of a physician decision-support system for diagnosis and management of mental disorders. A telepsychiatry unit in Maharashtra has reported on the feasibility and referral patterns.[9]

In this chapter we have deliberately chosen to use the term "telepsychiatry" to describe our program rather than the broader term "telemental health," as the services delivered under our program pertain to management/treatment of mental disorders, specifically psychoses, and the program largely functions as a psychiatric outpatient consultation service.

BACKGROUND

The Schizophrenia Research Foundation (SCARF) is a nongovernmental organization (NGO) that provides mental healthcare from its center in the southern city of Chennai, Tamil Nadu, India. As part of its community programs, SCARF has been operating outreach clinics in and around the city of Chennai for the past 30 years. SCARF substantially expanded the geographical coverage of its community outreach activities following the tsunami in 2004 by providing psychosocial support and training and running community clinics in two of the affected costal districts of Tamil Nadu.

SCARF's foray into telepsychiatry, funded initially by Oxfam Trust and subsequently by the Deutsche Bank Foundation, was aimed at assessing the feasibility of using telepsychiatry to provide psychosocial support and counseling for those affected by the tsunami disaster. SCARF operated as the central hub from which psychiatric support was provided to individuals who accessed care initially from two peripheral units, which connected to SCARF on a weekly basis. By the end of 3 years, the hub at SCARF Chennai was connected to seven peripheral units, where consultation was provided at regularly scheduled intervals that ranged from once a week at some sites to once a month at others, depending on patient load. The ISDN lines were chosen for the network as they were the most easily available and reliable. The peripheral units were located within the premises of local NGOs that in some instances had no prior experience in the delivery of healthcare services, let alone mental health. The teleclinics were run in conjunction with the staff of the local NGO who were trained in the basics of mental health by the SCARF community mental health team. Efforts to recruit a local physician into the process proved unsuccessful. This resulted in patients being referred to the nearest governmental hospital for a physical examination when needed. SCARF psychiatrists also periodically visited the peripheral units to have a face-to-face consultation with the more challenging cases.

This pilot project was successful, as it demonstrated that it was possible to deliver telepsychiatry services in remote villages that did not have formal mental health services. Since the required infrastructure and trained personnel were available, the logical next step was to expand the telepsychiatry services. This was seen as an ideal way to reach out to remote areas and conduct outreach clinics without unduly straining limited human resources. SCARF drew inspiration from the model it used in setting up community outreach programs in collaboration with local NGOs and used this as the template to set up its telemedicine service.[10]

Collaborating with a local NGO has multiple benefits, the primary advantage being its preexisting links with the local community and the availability of its grassroots-level workers drawn from the local population. These community level workers (CLWs) are familiar with the terrain, language, and customs of their region and, more importantly, have strong ties with the local community. Piggybacking onto their preexisting networks offers an excellent opportunity to scale down the cost of service provision.[11] The CLWs are trained to identify those in need of a psychiatric consultation and then refer them to the clinic. If the local NGO had the necessary infrastructure, the clinic could be established on their premises. See Box 6.1 for more information about CLWs.

SCARF TELEPSYCHIATRY IN PUDUKOTTAI

In 2010 the telepsychiatry program of SCARF was considerably expanded with support from the Tata Education Trust to cover the district of Pudukottai in Tamil Nadu. This district was chosen because it had one of

Box 6.1   COMMUNITY LEVEL WORKERS (CLWS)

Who are they?

- Hired from the local community and residing within the catchment area of the program.
- Recruited for attitude rather than knowledge base and experience.
- Not infrequently has a family member affected with a mental disorder
- Preferably young women with high school level of education.
- Women are preferred because they are seen as less threatening and can more easily gain entry into rural households especially if the ill individual is also a woman.

What are their responsibilities?

- Identifying and referring patients to the clinics.
- Creating awareness through folk music, street plays, skits, and other activities in keeping with the local culture and sensibilities.
- Screen patients at the clinic, collect basic history, facilitate the psychiatric consultation, dispense medication, and ensure follow-up of patients.
- Conducting psychoeducation, rehabilitation, adherence management; improving access to employment opportunities; and networking with community agencies for social inclusion.

What is their training?

- They attended a series of lectures and workshops on mental health disorders and psychosocial management.
- Trained on the basic instruments used for screening, collecting history, etc.
- Trained in conducting awareness programs.
- Ongoing training and supervision by psychiatric social worker.

What is the structure?

- The team of CLWs is managed by a qualified social worker who monitors their activities and provides professional supervision.
- The CLWs in turn work with volunteers and members of self-help group (SHG) clusters involved in microfinancing of livelihood activities that can facilitate the rehabilitation of the ill individuals within the community.
- As such the team is composed of a flexible group composed of a mental health professional), trained lay workers, volunteers, and preexisting SHGs.

the lowest social developmental indices in Tamil Nadu. The other major factor was the absence of mental health services under the public health-care system of the district.

It was decided to confine the project, SCARF Telepsychiatry in Pudukottai (STEP), to treating those with severe mental disorders, especially psychotic disorders. This was based on the fact that nonpharmacological treatments such as psychotherapy were difficult to implement over telepsychiatry[12] and were also resource intensive. The other factor guiding the decision was the effectiveness of pharmacological intervention as a first line treatment for psychotic disorders.

A survey of the catchment area revealed the prevalence of severe mental disorders (psychosis) to be 5 per 1000 population of whom 57% were currently untreated of whom nearly half (45%) have never been treated with the rest having discontinued treatment.[13]

Design and Structure of the Program

About 250 villages (population 500,000) were identified as the immediate catchment area of the program. The telepsychiatry peripheral clinics were to be started in four different areas to attain maximum geographical coverage of the district. The locations were selected based on the ease of access to them by the local population. The program was designed to serve about 1,500 patients in 3 years.

The hub-and-spoke model was used for the delivery of service. The peripheral units (spokes) were either fixed-line telepsychiatry clinics or mobile telepsychiatry clinics and connected to the hub at SCARF, Chennai. The fixed-line services were provided from two locations within the district catering to a population of 200,000, while the mobile service was provided in six locations covering a population of 300,000.

The teleclinics followed a weekly cycle. One of the major advantages of telepsychiatry is that only basic components (i.e., videoconferencing) are required compared with other specialties. For example, ophthalmology, oncology, or cardiology depend heavily on high-quality imaging data requiring sophisticated input devices such as digital ophthalmoscopes or electrocardiograms (ECGs) for diagnosis, which requires the necessary equipment to be available and functional at all times. The fact that only the videoconferencing equipment is required for telepsychiatry allows the teleclinics to continue functioning even in case of breakdown of equipment, as a laptop computer can be taken to the area and videoconferencing initiated using free software such as Skype, thus allowing the teleconsultation to take place as scheduled.

See Figure 6.1 for a detailed flow chart of activities pertaining to the program.

Fixed-Line Telepsychiatry

The fixed-line services were located within rented premises in villages in the catchment area and were equipped with integrated videoconferencing devices available commercially, which include a camera, microphone, data solution box (DSB), and flat panel display. It was a deliberate choice to go with a fully integrated unit, as this was seen as more rugged than a computer-based videoconferencing system, which had greater likelihood of operational failure in hot and dusty conditions. Static Internet protocol

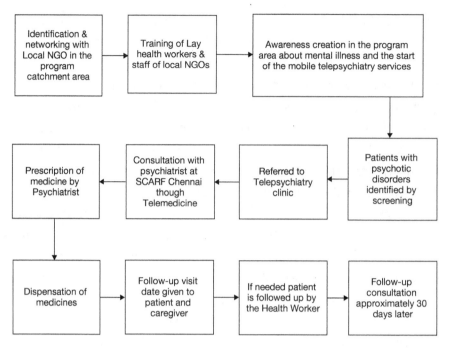

Figure 6.1 Flow chart indicating activities and the process that are followed.

on broadband Internet was chosen for network connectivity, as it was available and cost-effective.

Mobile Telepsychiatry

The mobile telepsychiatry service was mounted inside a specially designed bus with a private consultation chamber equipped with free videoconferencing software such as Skype loaded onto a laptop that connected through a wireless 3G broadband network to the central hub at Chennai. Initially other modes of connectivity were explored, including a very small aperture terminal (VSAT), but were dropped due to high cost. The bus also has a built in pharmacy from which the prescribed medicines are dispensed by a pharmacist. (This mobile telepsychiatry service is distinct from "mobile Health," which uses mobile phones to deliver healthcare services and is not discussed here.)

Awareness Programs

Prior to the start of the clinic, awareness programs were conducted in the villages about mental illness and the availability of the telepsychiatry service. These were also specifically designed to inform the local residents about telepsychiatry and the processes involved. A public address system and a large flat-screen television were fitted at the rear of the bus to screen educational films on mental health.

The awareness programs were conducted by CLWs in association with the local NGOs. This included street plays, lectures, or awareness videos at places where people gathered (workplaces during lunch breaks, marketplaces), and distribution of pamphlets. The local administration, village leaders, and local media were all informed of these initiatives.

Consultation and Treatment

Patients were identified and referred by CLWs to the telepsychiatry centers. Detailed assessments were done for all patients who were registered at these centers. The CLWs and nurses collected information on frequency of symptoms, duration, and so on, and also measured vital signs like weight, height, waist circumference, blood pressure, and pulse rate. This information was presented to the psychiatrist at SCARF in Chennai. The psychiatrist would then obtain a detailed clinical history and do a mental state examination. Following this a diagnosis was made and appropriate medicines prescribed. These medicines were dispensed at the pharmacy attached to the clinics.

To test the efficacy of this process, the Positive and Negative Syndrome Scale (PANSS)[14] was administered to a subset of 82 patients with schizophrenia at baseline and at the end of 1 year. It revealed that mean PANSS scores for the group fell from 80 (SD 28) to 47 (SD 25) at follow-up, demonstrating a significant reduction in psychopathology and the effectiveness of the treatment provided through telepsychiatry.[13]

As can be seen in Figure 6.2, while the stated objective of the program was to provide care to those with psychoses, the service ended up catering

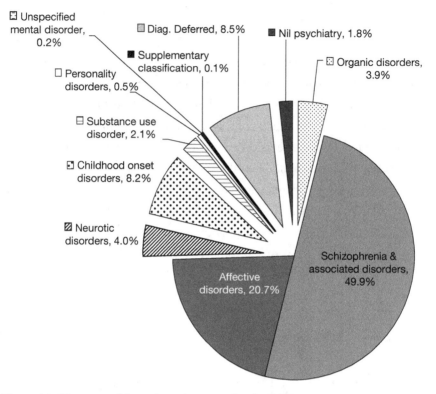

Figure 6.2 Diagnoses of the registered cases under the STEP program.

to a much wider range of disorders, with about 30% of patients having other diagnoses. This was primarily due to the fact that with no other affordable mental health services being available in the area it was impossible to turn away patients and families in acute distress.

Pharmacy

The provision of free medication was an essential component of the program, considering the patients' financial limitations and the fact that psychiatric drugs are rarely stocked in rural pharmacies. It was seen as imperative to provide as many components of the service under one roof as possible to encourage better use of service, leading to improved adherence to treatment and better outcomes.

Medical Records

Every registered patient was assigned a unique patient number. A standard patient dossier was created for each patient, and information on demographics, history of illness, mental status examination, level of functioning, and prescriptions were documented and updated after each visit. The patient records were maintained at both the hub in SCARF Chennai and at the peripheral unit. A computerized medical records system that was designed specifically for the program was used at the hub, while the peripheral units preferred to maintain paper records. This was essentially because the CLWs at the peripheral units were more comfortable in maintaining records in the local language, Tamil, and were not used to computers.

Each patient also receives a patient-held record designed to facilitate continuity of care and information sharing between healthcare professionals. It details their diagnosis, prescription, and any relevant investigations that the patient must get done independently, such as blood tests, and so forth.

Follow-Up and Reminders

The patients were followed up and reminded through phone calls (about 80% of patients/families have access to cell phones) about their scheduled clinic dates, and so forth. The implementation of this aspect of the service saw patient dropout rates reduce by over 50% over a period of 3 months.

All patients and families were also given an emergency contact number, which was manned around the clock 7 days a week. During emergencies, such as adverse reaction to medication or acute exacerbation of symptoms, the psychiatrist to whom the phone connects guided the family or the attending personnel in dealing with it.

Taking advantage of the wide availability of mobile phones in the community, some of the basic features available on most mobile phones were leveraged to improve follow-up rates at the clinic. These included programming them to ring alarms and provide reminders about the time for medication and follow-up visit dates.

Psychosocial Rehabilitation

Apart from identifying patients and referring them to the clinics, the CLWs also followed up the patients and delivered psychosocial rehabilitation (PSR) services. These PSR programs were run in coordination with local NGOs when possible. An important element was the formation of self-help groups (SHGs) that largely focused on economic activities. The families of the patients were also strongly encouraged to participate, since this helped to maintain continuity even if some patients relapsed or were unable to work.

Structured educational programs were also conducted for family members to help them better understand the illness and to enable them to manage it. They were also linked-up with local agencies and governmental departments that provide social benefits and services that they were entitled to receive.

Certification of disability was also done in coordination with the concerned department of the state government. These patients would now receive disability pension/benefits. This was a new initiative in that area. To date, about 10% of the registered patients have accessed disability benefits.

Cost of Service Provision

The average cost of service provision per patient per month was calculated as INR 694, approximately $US11. This is inclusive of consultation, medication for a month, at least one home visit by the CLW apart from one reminder call/contact, and establishment costs such as Internet charges, electricity and fuel costs, and so forth.

This costing is based only on recurrent expenditure and does not take into account the initial one-time investments made in terms of capital expenditure and infrastructure development that include videoconferencing equipment, computers, bus, awareness programs, initial training provided, development of the material, electronic medical records, and so forth.

While no direct comparable data is available regarding cost of service provision, reports from a public hospital from Delhi,[15] India, indicate that patients and their families spend anything ranging from INR 60 ($US1) to INR 520 ($US8) a month on medication alone for a severe mental disorder like schizophrenia. However, from the service provider's perspective, there is practically no published information on costs of consultation and other therapies.

Achievements of the STEP Program

This program has pioneered the use of mobile telepsychiatry in India. It has also been very efficient in getting the untreated, chronic mentally ill to treatment. Over 50% of this untreated group are now accessing our services.

The reach of the services extended well beyond the originally envisioned program area, with 45% of those seeking telepsychiatry services being from outside the program catchment area.

It was interesting to note that the reach of the mobile telepsychiatry clinics within the catchment area was greater, with about 61% of the patients within the area accessing these services, compared with the fixed-line clinics (49%). However, the fixed-line clinics had wider reach (more patients from outside the catchment area accessing the service) compared with the mobile clinics. And as such, overall registration at both types of clinics showed no difference in the number of beneficiaries.

The program also clearly demonstrated that telepsychiatry is effective in diagnosing and appropriately managing severe mental disorders. The fact that 1,500 patients had accessed care during a 3-year period also indicates that the service is acceptable and that patients and families are comfortable using it.

The use of mobile phones as a low-cost strategy to monitor patient follow-up and compliance has been initiated and will also be evaluated. It is premature to comment on its efficacy now.

The success of the program to a large extent is due to the availability and willingness of local NGOs and CLWs who were enthusiastic about participating in the delivery of mental health services even though they had no prior exposure. This level of task shifting is feasible and possible and more importantly essential for successful implementation of this type of program in the community.

Challenges Faced

Some of the challenges faced include lack of availability of network connectivity in the more rural isolated pockets, which were in greater need of services due their isolation and lack of access to health services.

The inconsistent availability of bandwidth leading to variable video quality was another challenge. This was resolved to some extent by muting the videoconferencing process (to reduce bandwidth use) and conducting the audio component over a phone.

Management of acutely ill persons who need to be hospitalized remains a challenge that has yet to be completely addressed.

It has also been challenging to impart more advanced PSR skills to the CLWs. While some family support and education were provided, intensive PSR inputs may well be beyond the scope of this initiative.

The management of physical comorbidity in patients, which is frequently present in economically disadvantaged and nutritionally compromised individuals, is another challenge. The project is trying to liaise with local general practitioners and the public health system for this.

Stigma related to mental illness is a challenge faced universally by health service providers across all models of service delivery. The lack of patronage of the mobile service by those from outside the catchment area could possibly be related to reluctance to be seen entering a bus (that is parked in a widely used public space for ease of access) that treats people with mental illness, versus the relative anonymity and privacy of the fixed-line clinic that sees greater usage by those from outside the catchment area. This appears not to be a deterrent for the local population, where the dictum "There are no secrets in a village" seems to operate. Creating some privacy for those waiting for the mobile service could yield improved usage.

CONCLUSION

India certainly needs a telemedicine act in place as well as a regulatory authority that will monitor and license users. It must however be enacted and enforced in such a manner that it will not hinder the progress of this technology, which could be the answer to the acute shortage of trained medical professionals that India faces.

It must be understood that telepsychiatry only redistributes resources and does not create additional capacity. It is essential to remember this when a telepsychiatry network is being initiated.

SCARF's experience with the program has been extremely positive. We strongly believe that running mobile telepsychiatry clinics in conjunction with CLWs trained in mental health in villages is an effective and replicable model of mental healthcare service delivery in resource-poor settings. With the recent emergence of improved and relatively cheap network technologies, this seems to be AN ideal time to exploit its immense potential.

ACKNOWLEDGMENT

The SCARF Telepsychiatry in Pudukottai (STEP) program was funded by Tata Education Trust of the Sir Dorabji Tata Trust and the Allied Trusts.

REFERENCE

1. World Health Organization. World health statistics 2012. Geneva: WHO, 2012.
2. Math SB, Srinivasaraju R. Indian psychiatric epidemiological studies: learning from the past. Indian Journal of Psychiatry. 2010;52(1):S95–S103.
3. Hyler SE, Gangure DP, Batchelder ST. Can telepsychiatry replace in-person psychiatric assessments? A review and meta-analysis of comparison studies. CNS Spectrums. 2005;10(5):403–413.
4. Ganapathy K. Telemedicine in the Indian context: an overview. Studies in Health Technology and Informatics. 2004;104:178–181.
5. Sood SP. Implementing telemedicine technology: lessons from India World hospitals and health services. 2004;40(3)29–30.
6. Indian Space Research Organisation (ISRO). Telemedicine healing touch through space enabling specialty healthcare to the rural and remote population of India. Publications and Public Relations Unit; ISRO HQ, Bangalore; 2005.
7. Sood SP. Telemedicine in India. Vol. 1. Government of India's Initiative. 2002.
8. Malhotra S, Chakrabarti S, Shah R, Gupta A, Mehta A, Nithya B, Kumar V, Sharma M. Development of a novel diagnostic system for a telepsychiatric application: a pilot validation study. BMC Research Notes. 2014;9(7):508.
9. Balasinorwala VP, Shah NB, Chatterjee SD, Kale VP, Matcheswalla YA. Asynchronous telepsychiatry in Maharashtra, India: study of feasibility and referral pattern. Indian Journal of Psychological Medicine. 2014;36:299–301.
10. Thara R, John S, Rao K. Telepsychiatry in Chennai, India: the SCARF experience. Behavioral Sciences & the Law. 2008;26(3):315–322.
11. Thara R, Padmavati R. A community mental health programme in rural Tamil Nadu. Asia Pacific Disability Rehabilitation Journal. 1999;10(1):34–36.
12. O'Reilly R, Bishop J, Maddox K, Hutchinson L, Fisman M, Takhar J. Is telepsychiatry equivalent to face-to-face psychiatry? Results from a randomized controlled equivalence trial. Psychiatric Services. 2007;58:836–843.
13. Venkatraman L, John S, Rao K, Thara R. Using telepsychiatry to bridge the mental health service gap in India. Presented during Royal College of Psychiatrists International Congress 2014. Abstract published 2014. http://www.rcpsych.ac.uk/pdf/Poster%20abstracts% 2005%2006%2014%20%282%29.pdf.
14. Kay SR, Fiszbein A, Opler LA. The Positive and Negative Syndrome Scale (PANSS) for schizophrenia. Schizophr Bulletin. 1987;13:261–269.
15. Sharma P, Das SK, Deshpande SN. An estimate of the monthly cost of two major mental disorders in an Indian metropolis. Indian Journal of Psychiatry. 2006;48(3):143–148.

7

Telemental Health Services in Sri Lanka

SISIRA EDIRIPPULIGE AND ROHANA B. MARASINGHE

S ri Lanka is an island nation with a population of 20.4 million (2013 census) located off the southeast coast of India. Of Sri Lanka's population, 77% live in rural areas and nearly a third of those employed work in the agriculture sector.[1] The health system of Sri Lanka consists of both public and private sector health service providers. The public sector plays a greater role in delivering health services to the population. Health services provided by the government-owned healthcare institutions are free of charge. According to World Bank estimates, in 2013, resources allocated to health services were 1.4% of the GDP of the country. Internationally, Sri Lanka claims to have some relatively better health indicators among developing countries such as low child and maternity mortality, high immunization rates, and high life expectancy.

MENTAL HEALTH SERVICES IN SRI LANKA

Mental health however, has been a cause for concern in Sri Lanka for long time. Mental health needs in Sri Lanka are probably as high as, if not higher than, those in other parts of the world. Suicide rates are among the highest globally. During the period between 1985 and 1989, for example, the national suicide rate for males was the second highest in the world.[2] Even though the rate has lowered over the years, Sri Lanka still has a high suicide rate and a high rate of self-harm.[3] According to reports, nearly 100,000 people attempt suicide every year in Sri Lanka.[4]

Studies have shown that extreme poverty, socioeconomic deprivation, war, violence, and natural disasters have put enormous pressure on mental health of the people in the country.[5] Studies carried out in tsunami-affected areas of the country have found that 40% of people living in those areas had common mental disorders (CMDs).[5] The World Health Organization (WHO) Country Office has estimated a 3% incidence of severe mental disorders among the population.[6]

In recent times, mental health has been identified as a priority and there is a growing interest to address mental health problems of the population. In 2007, a subnational mental health survey was commissioned by the Ministry of Health in Sri Lanka with the assistance of the World Bank Health Sector Development Project. Unfortunately, the outcome of the survey has not been published.

Regardless of growing interest in the sector, the access to mental health services is still limited. Public hospitals are the main providers of mental health services in the country. There are mental health wards within large government hospitals, which are based in urban areas. Private hospitals are also mainly located in urban centers, and large private hospitals have consultant psychiatrists and mental health staff available for a fee. The National Institute of Mental Health (NIMH), the largest hospital devoted to mental health in Sri Lanka, is based in the capital, Colombo.

KEY BARRIERS TO ACCESSING MENTAL
HEALTH SERVICES

In general, social stigma attached to mental health is cited as a significant barrier for accessing services. The issue of social stigma has been identified as a particularly serious one in Asian countries.[7,8] Studies have shown that people in Sri Lanka are reluctant to seek medical assistance due to social attitudes toward mental illness.[9,10]

The lack of mental health literacy among people has also been seen as an important barrier to wider use of mental health services. In general, people do not consider mental illness as a serious disease that needs medical assistance. Often mental health is dealt with by traditional healers. The lack of knowledge and understanding of the existence of mental diseases, their types, and the benefits of medical treatments has been identified as a significant barrier.[11]

A related issue is the lack of information available for people regarding mental health. From providers' perspective, the lack of ways to communicate important information with people is a key barrier. Undoubtedly, geography and distance as well as the constraints created by circumstances such as conflicts and disasters have kept people not only from accessing mental health services but also from being informed about them.[4]

Due to a range of reasons, no proper evaluation is carried out of the mental health of both urban and rural populations of the country on a regular basis. Therefore, the prevalence of undiagnosed mental health problem is a key issue. This is particularly relevant to rural communities and people living in war- and disaster-affected areas.[4]

Problems associated with health service delivery, such as the lack of mental health workforce and resources, have been identified as more serious barriers to providing appropriate services to the population. The mental health workforce in Sri Lanka is significantly small. According to recent estimates, there is one psychiatrist per 500,000 persons. There are no specialized psychiatric nurses in the country. A small proportion of general nurses undergoes some training relating to mental health.[4]

From the health system's perspective, the separation between mental health and primary care is considered to be a major setback.[12] Due to this, people living in rural areas have little or no access to mental health within the current healthcare system. It is important to note that 77% of Sri Lanka's population lives in rural or remote areas of the country.

The disparity of access to mental health services is another important feature. Nearly the entire mental health workforce is located in urban hospitals, making access to mental health services in rural and remote populations extremely difficult. Particularly, the people living in war-ravaged areas and areas where major disasters such as the 2004 tsunami took place, have little or no access to mental health services.[4] Additionally, the increased demand for services has put enormous pressure on the small mental health workforce of the country. Studies have found that mental health staff have extreme difficulties in providing services.[13]

As noted, greater attention has been paid to the mental health issues in recent times. A number of government and private organizations have addressed some key issues relating to providing mental health services to communities.[14] Recent Sri Lanka governments have promised to provide more funding to mental health services.[15] Attempts have been made to make structural changes to integrate mental health within the healthcare system by establishing community mental health services.[16,17] International organizations such as the WHO have played a role in improving mental health services on the island. For example, the WHO has been directly involved in the development of the National Policy and Strategic Framework for Prevention and Control of Chronic Non-Communicable Diseases, where mental health has been paid important attention.[18] The WHO has also been involved in a number of projects relating to the mental health of communities, particularly among those in postconflict areas in Sri Lanka (WHO–Sri Lanka, 2014).[19] There are also some important activities currently underway to improve the mental health workforce.[12]

Among the measures discussed, the use of information and communication technologies (ICTs) to promote mental health, widely known as telemental health, is making a noticeable appearance. Some telemental health activities are outlined here.

Telemental Health in Sri Lanka

Sri Lanka's health sector has been an early adopter of telemedicine.[20] Over the years, there have been a number of telemedicine projects to understand the value of technology use in delivering health services. Some projects have been supported by the public sector, while various local and overseas nongovernmental agencies have also been involved in the efforts. Although telemedicine has not been integrated into mainstream healthcare delivery of the country, clinicians, patients, and policymakers have been receptive to the concept.[20]

Efforts have also been made to use ICTs to deliver mental health services. Over the years, various online and telephone-based services have been used to provide emergency and nonemergency mental healthcare. Primarily, there have been two key priorities in telemental health efforts: (1) education of the general public regarding mental health and mental health services and (2) delivery of mental health services.

Education of the General Public

A number of projects have focused on disseminating relevant information to the population to raise awareness regarding mental health. Media such as websites, television, and social media are being used to propagate mental health information and educate general public regarding mental health. Some such initiatives are emerging from the government, while others have nongovernmental players. For example, public players such as the National Council of Mental health Sri Lanka (http://www.ncmh.lk/ncmh_council.htm), the Institute of Mental Health Sri Lanka (http://www.imhlk.com/) and the Sri Lanka Mental Health Foundation have initiated a number of activities to educate people and raise awareness regarding mental health. These establishments have used their websites as key tools in delivering important information to the public. In addition, public media such as national television, print media, and public seminars have been used in this regard. It is also important to note that these organizations have used social media such as Facebook to educate people about mental health.

The use of Web portals for disseminating information has been a key method. For example, the government-initiated Health Net (http://www.suwasariya.gov.lk) is a Web portal dedicated to providing valid health-related information to people. People can find information relating to mental health and relevant services on the Web portal. Generally these Web portals also provide individualized advice and guidance to patients for free. Patients can log on to the Web portal to ask their questions, and relevant medical health professionals provide answers with no cost. This has been one way in which people can access mental health professionals in recent times.

It is fair to say that there has been increased interest in telemental health in the country in the period following the tsunami of December 2014.[21] Undoubtedly, the lack of mental health workers and the difficulties in accessing affected communities created unique circumstances for which the country and the international players had to seek innovative solutions. Telemedicine in general, and telemental health in particular, has been identified as a valuable tool in disaster situations.[22] In the Sri Lankan context, telemental health was used to provide mental health services to communities immediately after the 2004 tsunami and then in an ongoing fashion.[23] Extreme geographical and climatic situations forced the services to seek new methods. The emergency and humanitarian action division of the WHO's South-East Asia Region Office was responsible for establishing healthcare services in the disaster-struck regions of the country. This project comes under the broad objectives of the Center for Public Service Communications (CPSC).[24] In terms of telemental health, satellite services were established due to lack of infrastructure and network. With the assistance of the South-East Asia Regional Disaster Health Information Network (SEARHIN), mental health services provided counseling support to people in the affected communities in the country by telemedicine. Sri Lankan health authorities and international collaborators also used videoconferencing facilities and the infrastructure established by the International Maritime Satellite Organisation (INMARSAT) during the disaster recovery period.[21]

The realization of the value of such methods may be one reason for this. For health services, telemental health has been shown to be a viable option for providing services. For local health authorities and health workers, the experience and expertise gained locally and from overseas during that period may have been an incentive and a driver for adopting telemental health. It is also noteworthy that ongoing severe mental health issues of people affected by the disaster may have been a reminder for policymakers and health services of the importance of mental health.

Since then, there have been a number of mental health services using technology to provide services to different groups in the country. Help lines have become a major tool in the country. Several help lines have been functioning in the country. They use various technologies to provide services, such as telephone, e-mail, and Web portals. One good example is the services provided by the CCC Foundation (http://cccfoundation.org.au/cccline/). The key objective of this program is to support people in crisis situations, to help them get back to their normal life and rebuild resilience to deal with challenges. Such help lines are dedicated to provide services in the field of domestic violence, family disputes, relationship problems, sexual abuse, psychiatric illness and disorders, drug and alcohol issues, and child abuse, to note just a few. Some of these help lines are supported by overseas partners financially or in other in-kind manners. For example, CCC Foundation has close links with Lifeline Australia, through which Australian partners provide training to counselors in Sri Lanka.

Another similar program is the Sahana project. The key function of this program is providing advice and counseling to people online. Using free and open source software (FOSS) application, Sahana has created a Web portal that provides mental health services in relief operations, recovery, and rehabilitation.[25-27] Few other similar services have reported their activities.[28]

Another project aimed to help people with suicide ideation using a mobile phone–based system. A randomized controlled study carried out to evaluate this project showed positive results.[29]

From a technology point of view, the services have used a number of different technologies. Table 7.1 summarizes the commonly used telemental services in Sri Lanka.

More popular technologies are telephone and other low-cost Internet-based tools. Help lines use either ordinary telephones on landlines or mobile phones. These services provide emergency mental health services, and the majority of inquiries are related to suicide/self-harm prevention.

The other common method used in obtaining telemental services is short message service (SMS) messages. A number of help lines use SMS for providing services. The system is becoming popular, as the cost of SMS is low and the service can be used as an alternative way of contacting with therapists.

A review of randomized controlled trial evidence on telehealth approaches to suicide prevention revealed that telehealth approaches were

TABLE 7.1 CLASSIFICATION OF TELEMENTAL HEALTH SERVICE

	Real-Time	Store-and-Forward
Simple/ Less expensive	Voice telephone calls and hotlines[25–28,30]	SMS, e-mail, access to voice recording[29,31,32]
	– counseling services using Sahana project and CCC (Courage-Compassion-Commitment) project	– SMS-based study for helping people with suicide ideation
Complex/ More expensive	Video consultation, virtual world and live chat rooms	Web pages and databases[25–27] – Information delivery through websites such as CCC (Courage-Compassion-Commitment project and Sahana project

effective when the intervention was based on psychotherapies such as cognitive-behavioral therapy and problem-solving therapy. Notably, telephony has been used in most telehealth suicide-prevention approaches.[30]

It is important to note that there is an increasing tendency to use mobile devices, particularly mobile phones, for providing mental health services in the country.[31] One study has reported that the use of mobile phones for providing mental health service to clients was feasible and well accepted.[32] Fast-growing mobile phone use in Sri Lanka makes it a sensible method to use for health delivery, especially mental health services. This use of mobile devices in healthcare is known as mHealth.

Globally, mHealth is gaining popularity. A number of studies have shown the value using mHealth for mental health in developing countries.[33,34] The logic behind this tendency is that both clinicians and patients tend to use the most accessible technology for the need. Brian and Ben-Zeev (2014) showed that mHealth is playing an increasing role in Asia. Their study showed that mHealth can promote mental health literacy, provide greater access to mental health services, and support self-management of illness of people in Asia.[35]

CONCLUSIONS

This chapter reveals that the use of more complex and expensive telemedicine methods such as video-based consultations in mental health is still rare in Sri Lanka. As in other developing countries, the cost of and access to appropriate infrastructure are key constraints in using such advanced technologies in health service delivery.

Telemental health is a logical extension of striving to provide services to the population in the country. Healthcare providers and policymakers have realized the value of telemental health as a useful tool. A number of attempts are being made. More accessible and low-cost solutions have been the preferred options so far. Challenges such as lack of technology, appropriate infrastructure, knowledge, and skills are still key barriers for using this tool widely.[36]

REFERENCES

1. Department of Census and Statistics. Sri Lanka Labour Force Survey. 2014.
2. Vecchia C, Lucchini F, Levi F. Worldwide trends in suicide mortality, 1955–1989. Acta Psychiatrica Scandinavica. 1994;90(1):53–64.
3. de Silva VA, Senanayake S, Dias P, Hanwella R. From pesticides to medicinal drugs: time series analyses of methods of self-harm in Sri Lanka. Bulletin of the World Health Organization. 2012;90(1):40–46.
4. Siva N. Sri Lanka struggles with mental health burden. Lancet. 2010;375(9718): 880–881.
5. Catani C, Jacob N, Schauer E, Kohila M, Neuner F. Family violence, war, and natural disasters: a study of the effect of extreme stress on children's mental health in Sri Lanka. BMC Psychiatry. 2008;8(1):33.
6. Neuner F, Schauer E, Catani C, Ruf M, Elbert T. Post-tsunami stress: a study of posttraumatic stress disorder in children living in three severely affected regions in Sri Lanka. 2006.
7. Ng CH. The stigma of mental illness in Asian cultures. Australian and New Zealand Journal of Psychiatry. 1997;31(3):382–390.
8. Saraceno B, van Ommeren M, Batniji R, et al. Barriers to improvement of mental health services in low-income and middle-income countries. Lancet. 2007;370(9593):1164–1174.
9. Fernando SM, Deane FP, McLeod HJ. Sri Lankan doctors' and medical undergraduates' attitudes towards mental illness. Social Psychiatry and Psychiatric Epidemiology. 2010;45(7):733–739.
10. Khan MM. Suicide on the Indian subcontinent. Crisis. 2002;23(3):104.
11. Kotalawala S. EPA-0127–Health seeking behaviour in parents of children and adolescents with mental health problems in Sri Lanka. European Psychiatry. 2014;29:1.
12. Jenkins R, Mendis J, Cooray S, Cooray M. Integration of mental health into primary care in Sri Lanka. Mental Health in Family Medicine. 2012;9(1):15.
13. Lopes Cardozo B, Sivilli TI, Crawford C, et al. Factors affecting mental health of local staff working in the Vanni region, Sri Lanka. Psychological Trauma. 2013;5(6):581.
14. Javed M. Programs of mental health and policies in South Asia: origin and current status. In: Trivedi, Jitendra Kumar and Tripathi, Adarsh (Eds.), Mental Health in South Asia: Ethics, Resources, Programs and Legislation. Springer; 2015:81–94.
15. Commers M, Morival M, Devries M. Toward best-practice post-disaster mental health promotion for children: Sri Lanka. Health Promotion International. 2012;29(1):165–170. doi:10.1093/heapro/das047.
16. Ranasinghe P, Mendis J, Hanwella R. Community psychiatry service in Sri Lanka: a successful model. Sri Lanka Journal of Psychiatry. 2011;2(1):3–5.
17. Weerasundera R. Community psychiatry in a Sri Lankan setting: should we rush to push the boundaries? Sri Lanka Journal of Psychiatry. 2010;1(2):27–28.
18. Ministry of Healthcare and Nutrition Sri Lanka. National policy and strategic framework for prevention and control of chronic non-communicable diseases, 2009.
19. WHO–Sri Lanka. Country cooperation strategy at a glance. 2014. http://www.who.int/countryfocus/cooperation_strategy/ccsbrief_lka_en.pdf. Accessed July 2015.

20. Marasinghe RB, Edirippulige S, Smith AC, Abeykoon P, Jiffry MT, Wootton R. A snapshot of e-health activity in Sri Lanka. Journal of Telemedicine and Telecare. 2007;13(Suppl 3):53–56.

21. Scupola A, Gogia SB. Providing telemental health services after disasters: a case based on the post-tsunami experience. IGI Global; 2009.

22. Llewellyn CH. The role of telemedicine in disaster medicine. Journal of Medical Systems. 1995;19(1):29–34.

23. Vermetten E, Middelkoop CV, Taal L, Carll EK. Online psychotrauma intervention in the aftermath of the tsunami: a community-building effort. In: Elizabeth K. Carll (Ed.), Trauma psychology: issues in violence, disaster, health, and illness. Westport, CT: Praeger; 2007:255–271.

24. CPSC. Center for Public Service Communications. http://www.cpsc.com/index. php/our-work/health-information-and-technology. Accessed July 2015.

25. Careem M, De Silva C, De Silva R, Raschid L, Weerawarana S, eds. Sahana: Overview of a disaster management system. 2006 International Conference on Information and Automation (ICIA); 2006: IEEE.

26. Waidyanatha N, Gow G, Sampath C, et al., eds. Sahana alerting software for real-time biosurveillance in India and Sri Lanka. 2010 International Conference on Computer and Information Application (ICCIA); 2010: IEEE.

27. Yu Q, Wang Y, Chen X, Wu Y, eds. The emergency relief prototype system design and implementation based on LBS. International Conference on Management and Service Science, 2009 (MASS'09); 2009: IEEE.

28. Chapman KR, Arunatileka SM, eds. Teleconsultation roadmap: the path to tele-medicine. 2010 International Conference on e-Health Networking Applications and Services (Healthcom), 12th IEEE; 2010: IEEE.

29. Marasinghe RB, Edirippulige S, Kavanagh D, Smith A, Jiffry MT. Effect of mobile phone–based psychotherapy in suicide prevention: a randomized controlled trial in Sri Lanka. Journal of Telemedicine and Telecare. 2012;18(3):151–155.

30. Marasinghe RB. Telehealth-bringing healthcare to one's doorstep: how ready is Sri Lanka? Sri Lanka Journal of Bio-Medical Informatics. 2010;1(3):124–138.

31. Vatsalan D, Arunatileka S, Chapman K, et al., eds. Mobile technologies for enhancing eHealth solutions in developing countries. Second International Conference on eHealth, Telemedicine, and Social Medicine, 2010 (ETELEMED'10); 2010: IEEE.

32. Perera I. Implementing healthcare information in rural communities in Sri Lanka: a novel approach with mobile communication. Journal of Health Informatics in Developing Countries. 2009;3(2).

33. Mechael PN. The case for mHealth in developing countries. Innovations. 2009;4(1): 103–118.

34. Tomlinson M, Rotheram-Borus MJ, Swartz L, Tsai AC. Scaling up mHealth: where is the evidence? 2013.

35. Brian RM, Ben-Zeev D. Mobile health (mHealth) for mental health in Asia: objectives, strategies, and limitations. Asian Journal of Psychiatry. 2014;10:96–100.

36. Edirippulige S, Rohana B, Marasinghe VH, Abeykoon P, Wootton R. Eight strategies to promote e-health and telemedicine activities in developing countries. Telehealth in the Developing World. 2009:79.

8

Telemental Health in Taiwan

HSIU-HSIN TSAI

The Republic of China (Taiwan) is 36,000 square kilometers, encompassing the mainland islands of Taiwan and its offshore islands. On the Taiwan mainland, three-quarters of the land area is mountainous, with the majority of the mountains being more than 3,000 meters high. The unique geographic characteristics of Taiwan result in limited accessibility to healthcare services and less medical resources for rural (mountainous and isolated island area) residents, who are less likely to get comprehensive medical care. Telemedicine thus offers a possibility of resolving the issue of unequally distributed medical resources in Taiwan. In 1995 the Taiwan government officially launched a telemedicine program under the National Information Infrastructure (NII) project in an attempt to address this issue.[1] However, the National Health Insurance (NHI) system and other health policies in Taiwan limit the applicability of telemedicine in Taiwan, based on the laws of physicians (Article 11):

> A physician may not treat, issue prescription or certificate of diagnosis to patient not diagnosed by the physician himself or herself. In mountain areas, on outlying islands, in remote areas, or under special or urgent circumstances, however, and in response to medical needs, physician appointed by the competent authority in a special municipality or county (city) may use telecommunications methods to inquire about illness, set diagnosis and issue prescriptions, and treatment may be dispensed by nursing or obstetrics personnel belonging to health organizations.[1]

The diagnosis and treatment formulated in the previous item, the related treatment items, appointment of physician, and telecommunications methods are defined by the competent central authority. Therefore, the laws in Taiwan restrict the application of telemedicine in mountainous areas, outlying islands, and remote areas, hence limiting the development of telemedicine.

Furthermore, in 1995 the Taiwan government launched the NHI system, a compulsory social insurance program, which affects the applicability of telemedicine. Currently, telemedicine can be paid for by the NHI only in some situations. Based on the laws described, NHI only pays physicians who meet its criteria and regulations. Thus, in terms of outpatient payment, a physician will only be paid if he (she) has filed for support from NHI in advance.

The implementation of the telemedicine network in Taiwan has progressed through four stages: the initiation research stage (1994–1996), promotion research stage (1997–1999), application research stage (2000–2006), and the application stage (2007–present).[1]

In the initiation research stage, the government mainly funded distance education and teleconsultation experimental projects under the NII. There are four large-scale medical hospitals recruited under the telemedicine pilot program. Based on their characteristics (e.g., location and type of hospital), each of these large hospitals are arranged to be affiliated with hospitals in rural areas in order to carry out the telemedicine program. Services offered include patient assessment, remote diagnosis, and diagnostic or therapeutic consultation services across a wide array of specialty areas. Different bandwidths (ATM DS3, DSI, ISDN 128 K-384K) for different purposes (real-time consultation or education) were tested at this stage. Approximately 2,000 consultations are made every year using 1.5 Mbps bandwidth (half is used for videoconferencing while the other half is used for digital transmission in asynchronous consultation). Overall teleradiology is the most commonly used service.

In the promotion stage (1997–1999), applications in different medical disciplines were tested to promote multipoint videoconference and electronic journals. At this stage, the teleconsultation system had been applied to more than 10 medical subspecialties. Furthermore, the connection between two telemedicine centers in Taiwan was also tested at this stage. The delivery of telecourses to community hospitals via a videoconferencing system and the preliminary Internet continuing medical education network were also tested at this stage.

In 1999, Taiwan suffered the 921 earthquake, which occurred in Jiji, a mountainous area in Taiwan. This caused the government to focus on the development of telemedicine in mountainous areas in the next stage (application research stage, 2000–2006). This allowed large hospitals to cooperate with local primary centers in mountainous areas via telemedicine. Such services were helpful to the villages, which had a significant lack of medical doctors.

In order to address the long-term needs of the growing elderly population, the Ministry of Health and Welfare commissioned in 2007 the Telecare Pilot Project, which marked the start of the application stage (2007–now). A multidisciplinary team, comprising the medical equipment, information and communication technologies, and security sectors, was established to provide comprehensive health services. The team's objective is to develop a comprehensive telecare service model that covers the community-, home-, and institutional-based services.

The telecare service model consists of the following five services:

1. Teleconsultation: Using telecommunications equipment, residents consult healthcare professionals with regard to their sickness or ailments.

2. Telemonitoring: The data on patients' physiological
    measurements (e.g., blood pressure, body temperature,
    oxygen level, and blood glucose level) will be stored and
    interpreted. Based on these data, the hospital will provide
    reminder, care, and tracking management services.
3. Telecommunication: With coordination between family members
    and the nursing home, residents can communicate with their
    family members via telecommunication equipment.
4. Telesupervision: Though telecommunication equipment,
    healthcare professionals in hospitals can educate or exchange
    knowledge with nursing home staffs on healthcare.
5. Pharmaceutical services: Pharmacists and specialists can
    provide information on the prescription of drugs and their
    safety standards. They can also ensure the safety of residents
    through their professional judgments on repeated drug use
    and the substitutability of drugs.

TELEMENTAL HEALTH IN TAIWAN

A majority of psychiatrists reside in large cities and work in large-scale medical centers in Taiwan. Taiwan residents who want to be covered under the NHI have the option of choosing any hospital under this program for the treatment of their illnesses. Because large-scale hospitals have more advanced medical resources, most residents prefer going to these hospitals for medical treatment. This is evident in the fact that the largest medical center in Taiwan treats more than 10,000 outpatients per day while the average number of outpatients in other areas is merely 829 per day.[2] Patients may experience a longer waiting time during their visits to these hospitals, and might be especially hesitant to make such a visitation if they suffer from certain mental health problems, such as agoraphobia (anxiety related to leaving their homes) which prevents them from seeking treatment in hospitals. This is an example of how telemental health may offer a possibility to solve these problems.

Providing mental illness diagnoses using "Internet consultation and telecare" for mental health patients has been reported in Taiwan. During Internet consultations, instruments such as the depression scale are used as screening tools instead of diagnostic tools. There are several private mental health clinics carrying out Internet consultations in Taiwan, with the main form being webpages, e-mail, and message boards.[3] Patients can make appointments to have Internet consultations with their psychiatrists. However, this is not covered by the NHI and patients have to pay out-of-pocket for the full medical expense. In Internet consultations, counselors interact via a website with patients. The research done by Li and his colleagues,[4] showed comparable working alliance between Internet and face-to-face consultations. Although Internet consultation is regarded as having promising future prospects, its main problems are the lack of in-service training for Internet consulting agencies, practicum ethical guidelines, computer programs, and creation of work teams.[3]

As for telecare, institutional care services are one of the main areas of the telecare program. In some mental health institutions (or hospitals) residents with symptoms of mental illness may use the telemental system to obtain follow-up assessment and psychopharmacological management. Patients are first required to be assessed and diagnosed by a psychiatrist in person before using the telemental system. During the face-to-face assessment (which usually lasts 1.5 hours) both a psychiatrist and a psychologist are present. Medications are prescribed after a diagnosis is made. Consecutive medication prescriptions for chronic mental disease are limited to a quantity for up to 30 days treatment per time. The same psychiatrist who did the first evaluation can proceed to do telemental health assessments via videoconferencing for subsequent treatments.

VIDEOCONFERENCING TELEMENTAL HEALTH PROGRAM FOR THE ELDERLY: AN EXAMPLE

As in many countries, Taiwan faces an aging population, in which the percentage of elderly persons has increased to 11.84% in 2014.[5] Longer life span, low birth rate, smaller families, and urbanization have contributed to the increase in the number of elderly living in nursing homes. Nursing home placement has been widely discussed in the literature as a stressful life event that challenges older people. Moreover, the rapid growth of the nursing home population will arguably create problems for healthcare professionals. Depression is the most burdensome and prevalent mental illness among nursing home residents. The prevalence of depression among nursing home residents varied from 21% to 45% in Western countries and 45.7% to 81.8% in Taiwan.[6] In addition, many nursing home residents also experience loneliness.

Providing social support to the elderly is important, as the quality and quantity of social support systems used by older people are closely related to both their health status and quality of life. Most nursing home residents become functionally dependent due to their poor physical health, yet their psychosocial needs should not be neglected. One important aspect of social support for older nursing home residents is the continuous involvement of their family members. Research has demonstrated that when families are involved in the care plans of an institution, the residents, families, and staffs will benefit greatly from such interventions. However, it is reported that one-third of nursing home residents rarely had visitors. About 45%–60% of the residents' families visit them once a week.[7] A longitudinal study also revealed that the duration of these visits decreased 1.34 hours yearly. Fortunately, social support is not limited to only in-person visits.

Although family members may not visit the residents frequently due to time constraints, interactions over the phone may reduce residents' loneliness.[8] Nevertheless, human communications are rich in both verbal and nonverbal elements. Nonverbal communication can facilitate the establishment of mutual connection and understanding between the elderly residents and their families. With rapid advancements in technology, real-time audiovisual systems can serve as a form of telecommunication for nursing home residents who lack the skills and capacities to adapt to the nursing home environment.[9,10] Current telecommunication technology, such as videoconferencing, provides alternative means for elderly living in nursing home to interact with others. Videoconferencing has a positive impact on interpersonal interaction[11] and has been recognized as a feasible way of delivering care to frail elders with chronic diseases[8] and promoting social interactions among people with difficulties in communication.[12] These programs enable people with communication problems to use pictures and other media to share information about themselves.[13] Hence, these researches have proven the feasibility of videoconferencing as a communication platform for individuals living in institutions.

The videoconferencing program piloted in Taiwan by the author and colleagues, used laptops and Internet communication programs.[7,14,15] Nursing home residents were requested to use the program at least once a week, with the help of a trained research assistant, who spent at least 5 minutes per week with each resident for the first 3 months during their scheduled videoconference visits. The videoconferencing program was carried out weekly to reflect the frequency of in-person visits to a nursing home resident for the majority of families,[16] while the 3-month adjustment allowed residents to become familiar with the new videoconferencing program. After the 3-month adjustment period, residents who wanted to participate in the program and videoconference with their families were assisted by trained nursing home staff (nurses or nurses' aides). The residents mainly communicated with their child, grandchild, or significant other.

The communication applications used were Microsoft Network Video Conversation (MSN) or Skype via a 2M/256K wireless modem using a large screen (15.6-inch) laptop. Laptops were left in the nursing homes for 1 year. All residents in both the intervention and comparison groups completed questionnaires for demographic information (baseline only), depressive symptoms, loneliness, and social support at baseline as well as at 3, 6, 9, and 12 months.

Qualitative Outcome of the Program

At the end of the 3-month videoconferencing program, the participants were interviewed in person with semistructured questionnaires to understand their experiences of using videoconference communication with their families in the nursing home. The questionnaires include questions as follows: "Are you satisfied with the program? What impressed you the most when using the videoconference to communicate with your family? What are the differences between in person visit and videoconference visit?" Participants (average age 75.4, range 60–95) reported being appreciative of the videoconferencing program and believed it to be worthy of promotion. They were very grateful to have this activity, which narrowed the gap between them and their families. The average duration of each videoconference communication was 11.75 minutes. Participants' subjective perceptions of using videoconferencing were described in four major themes: enriched life (100%), second-best option for visiting (62.5%), life adjustments (50%), and true picture of family life (32.5%).[14]

Quantitative Outcome of the Program

Furthermore, we evaluated both short-term and long-term quantitative effects of our programs.[7,15] Data were collected four times (baseline, 3 months, 6 months, and 12 months) through face-to-face interviews regarding social support, loneliness, and depressive status using the Social Supportive Behavior Scale, University of California Los Angeles Loneliness Scale, and Geriatric Depression Scale respectively. The Social Supportive Behavior Scale evaluated residents based on the four dimensions of social support behavior (emotional, informational, instrumental, and appraisal support) as well as the number of family members or friends who contacted residents and the number of contacts (either by phone or in person) during the previous week. Although 55% of our experimental group do visit the nursing home residents at least once a week, they still used videoconferencing as a way to contact residents when they are unable to visit the residents in person.[15]

Our study has demonstrated that videoconference intervention alleviated elderly nursing home residents' perceived loneliness and improved their depressive status 3, 6, and 12 months after the intervention. The changes in depression scores (GDS) were on average significantly lower in the experimental group than the changes in the comparison group at 3, 6, or 12 months (β = −2.64, −4.33, and −4.40, respectively, with all p values < .010) (Table 8.1). This might be due to videoconference providing a "social presence" to older adults.[17] Future studies may include a control group to demonstrate efficacy of this intervention. For elderly residents in nursing homes, videoconferencing might add color to their lives. Thus, our results suggest that videoconferencing is a good way to reduce loneliness of the elderly in both the community and institutions.

Our research showed that videoconferencing had no effects on instrumental social support at the 3-month data collection time, as previously reported.[18] However, we found that instrumental social support decreased significantly over time, but not the number of family members' in-person visits. In other words, although family members continue to visit the

TABLE 8.1 EFFECTS OF VIDEOCONFERENCE INTERVENTION ON PARTICIPANTS' DEPRESSIVE STATUS AND LONELINESS AT 3, 6, AND 12 MONTHS IN CONSIDERATION OF TIME × GROUP EFFECTS

Variable	Unadjusted				Adjusted[a]			
	β	SE	χ^2	p	β	SE	χ^2	p
Depressive status								
Time × Group[b]								
3 months × group[b]	−1.36	.56	5.97	.02	−2.64	.57	21.31	<.001
6 months × group[b]	−4.50	.97	21.64	<.001	−4.33	1.03	17.59	<.001
12 months × group[b]	−4.45	.89	24.91	<.001	−4.40	.92	23.13	<.001
Loneliness								
Time × Group[b]								
3 months × group[b]	−4.84	1.14	17.95	<.001	−5.40	1.22	19.62	<.001
6 months × group[b]	−6.46	1.64	15.42	<.001	−6.47	1.70	14.47	<.001
12 months × group[b]	−6.42	1.64	15.34	<.001	−6.27	1.94	10.50	.001

[a] Adjusted for residents' age and length of residency
[b] Group 0: comparison group, Group 1: experimental group

elderly residents in person, they provided less instrumental social support in terms of specific items and assistance. After a long stay in a nursing home, elderly residents tend to adapt to the environment and hence do not need extra items for their daily lives, which might be one possible reason for this finding.

It is interesting that when asked, family members reported low acceptance of desktop-based videoconferencing (13.5%–28.6%). This was due to inability to use videoconference technology as well as the lack of appropriate equipment, such as computers.[7,15] However, these barriers may no longer be applicable in current situations due to greater availability of relatively inexpensive communication devices such as mobile phones and tablets.[19,20]

Furthermore, our results showed that the use of videoconference visits decreased over time. This decreased use of videoconferencing was likely due to a loss in the novelty of videoconferencing, lack of staff to help the residents operate the devices, a need to remind family members to use videoconferencing, and some residents running out of things to say during videoconferences. Owing to the emphasis on the balance of relationships within groups in the Chinese culture, Chinese are more hesitant about taking the initiative in conversations. Hence, this results in the loss of conversation topics between residents and their family members. Added to this tendency is the novelty of videoconference interactions, particularly for older adults, which might inhibit their natural ability to start a discussion.

RECOMMENDATIONS FOR APPLICATION OF VIDEOCONFERENCING IN ELDERLY POPULATIONS

At the outset of our study, many elderly participants were concerned about having no prior experience in using the computer or having limited computer capabilities. However, it was shown that the ability of older adults to use computers can be enhanced through appropriate training,[21] and even older adults with dementia can be trained to use computers.[22] In addition, older adults were found to be eager to learn computer skills, as it gives them a sense of personal control. However, some elderly possess physical limitations such as visual or hearing impairment, hence appropriate equipment may be necessary to assist them in minimizing or overcoming these limitations. Furthermore, we also suggested that more interactive content could be developed for videoconferencing to increase the length of videoconferencing use.

CHALLENGES FACING THE FUTURE
FOR TELEMENTAL HEALTH IN TAIWAN

Although telemental health provides a convenient medical resource in Taiwan, the lack of human touch is one of the challenges of its application. Human touch is an important component of in-person treatment behavior that provides mental support in disease treatment in Taiwan. In addition, the restrictive laws in Taiwan do not allow for broader implementations of telemedicine. Currently, there is no association that promotes telemedicine in Taiwan or influences government's policymaking decisions in this area. Furthermore, the transmission of medical data may have accuracy, safety, and other technological issues. There is no related law focusing on telemedicine, electronic signatures, and patient privacy protection. Accidents due to medical negligence are usually attributed to two factors—physicians' poor choice of treatment methods which may be done out of obligation, and invasive medical procedures that worsened patients' medical conditions. In the case of medical negligence in telemedicine, there is the issue of whether suing the consulted physician, a third party, will cause any tensions in the doctor–patient relationship. In this case, the following questions must be taken into consideration: Can the harms to the plaintiff be foreseen? Is there a close causal relationship between the harm experienced by the plaintiff and the defendant's actions? What are the ethical responsibilities of the defendant's actions? Are there any policies to prevent future harm? Can the risks be covered by insurance? Due to legal uncertainties, there are problems with medical malpractice liability. For instance, there is the issue of whether physicians can diagnose and prescribe medication through videoconferencing. Current laws in Taiwan also do not explicitly address the issues that may arise due to the limitations of telemedicine. For example, when a physician (located at place A) diagnoses a patient (located at place B), what should the location of diagnosis be? Who is the superintendent of government? Who will charge the illegal behavior for the jurisdiction (place A or B)?

Additionally, health insurance usually does not cover expenditures on telemedicine and telemental health services. This represents a major economic burden for patients, as they have to pay for the full cost. If telemedicine is paid by health insurance, the issue of physician resistance, an important bottleneck to the adoption and diffusion of telemedicine in healthcare, may also be solved. The lack of technological infrastructure, quality equipment, and allocated budget does not allow hospitals in remote and rural areas to provide telemental health services. Privacy issues arise as challenges to expanding telemental health services in Taiwan. As data are being stored electronically, unauthorized access to highly sensitive medical information may occur. Thus, regulatory standards for privacy protection should be established. This should include confidentiality issues on telecommunications, a standard or criteria for the access to patients' personal information by third parties, restrictions on the database, and the exceptions made during emergency situations or when patients are comatose.

Finally, although the telehealth systems and services in Taiwan are developed based on the research outcome, there is a lack of standardization of telehealth system components and services. Currently, health professionals do not undergo any special training that not only allows them to understand telehealth better but also promotes the efficiency of telehealth systems. However, trainings should not be confined only to technology use and operations but also, when appropriate, should include verbal communication and detection of important nonverbal expressions or cues in a virtual setting. Preserving professional authority and autonomy in telemedicine services is also important.

REFERENCES

1. Chen HS. Telemedicine. In: Cheng HL, ed. Medical information management. 2nd ed. Taipei, Taiwan: Farseeing; 2013:639–646.
2. Ministry of Health and Welfare. The statistics analysis of medical care institution's status & hospital's utilization, 2012. http://www.mohw.gov.tw/cht/DOS/Statistic_P.aspx?f_list_no=312&fod_list_no=5126&doc_no=46170. Published August 19, 2014. Accessed July 19, 2015.
3. Wang CH, Lin CW, Liu SH, Yang CF, Hsiao EL. A survey study on development of cybercounseling in Taiwan. Bulletin of Educational Psychology. 2008;39(3):395–412.
4. Li WP, Chen CF, Wang CH. Agreements on working alliance and session impact in cybercounseling and interview counseling. Bulletin of Education Psychology. 2008;40(1):1–22.
5. Ministry of Interior. Interior statistic. http://statis.moi.gov.tw/micst/stmain.jsp?sys=100. Accessed July 19, 2015.
6. Huang HT, Chuang YH, Hsueh YH, Lin PC, Lee BO, Chen CH. Depression in older residents with stroke living in long-term care facilities. Journal of Nursing Research. 2014;22(2):111–118.
7. Tsai HH, Tsai YF, Wang HH, Chang YC, Chu HH. Videoconference program enhances social support, loneliness, and depressive status of elderly nursing home residents. Aging and Mental Health. 2010;14:947–954.
8. Hine N, Arnott JL. A multimedia social interaction service for inclusive community living: initial user trials. University Access Information Society. 2002;2:8–17.
9. Hui E, Woo J, Hjelm M, Zhang YT, Tsui HT. Telemedicine: a pilot study in nursing home residents. Gerontology. 2001;47(2):82–87.
10. Nakamura K, Takano T, Akao C. The effectiveness of videophones in home healthcare for the elderly. Medical Care. 1999;37:117–125.
11. Finn KE, Sellen AJ, Wibur SB. Video-mediated communication. Mahwah, NJ: Routledge; 1997.
12. Keck CS, Doarn CR. Telehealth technology applications in speech-language pathology. Journal of Telemedicine and E-health. 2014;20(7):653–659.
13. Nilsen LL. Collaborative work by using videoconferencing: opportunities for learning in daily medical practice. Qualitative Health Research. 2011;21:1147–1158.
14. Tsai HH, Tsai YF. Older nursing home residents' experiences with videoconferencing to communicate with family members. Journal of Clinical Nursing. 2010;19(11–12):1538–1543.
15. Tsai HH, Tsai YF. Changes in depressive symptoms, social support and loneliness over 1 year after a minimum 3-month videoconference program for older nursing home residents. Journal of Medical Internet Research. 2011;13(4):e93.
16. Port CL, Gruber-Baldini AL, Burton L, et al. Resident contact with family and friends following nursing home admission. Gerontologist. 2001;41(5):589–596.

17. Cukor P, Baer L, Willis BS, et al. Use of videophones and low-cost standard tele-phone lines to provide a social presence in telepsychiatry. Telemedicine Journal. 1998;4(4):313–321.

18. Walther JB, Park MR. Cues filtered out, cues filtered in: computer-mediated com-munication and relationships. In: Knapp ML, Daly JA, eds. Handbook of interper-sonal communication. Thousand Oaks, CA: Sage; 2002:529–563.

19. Demiris G, Afrin LB, Speedie S, et al. Patient-centered applications: use of informa-tion technology to promote disease management and wellness. A white paper by the AMIA knowledge in motion working group. Journal of the American Medical Informatics Association. 2008;15(1):8–13.

20. Tak SH, Benefield LE, Mahoney DF. Technology for long-term care. Research in Gerontological Nursing. 2010;3(1):61–72.

21. Dauz E, Moore J, Smith CE, Puno F, Schaag H. Installing computers in older adults' homes and teaching them to access a patient education web site: a systematic approach. Computers, Informatics, Nursing. 2004;22:266–272.

22. Malcolm M, Mann WC, Tomita MR, Fraas LF, Stanton KM, Gitlin L. Computer and Internet use in physically frail elders. Physical and Occupational Therapy in Geriatrics. 2001;19:15–32.

9

Telemental Health Services for Indigenous Communities in Australia

A Work in Progress?

SISIRA EDIRIPPULIGE, MATTHEW BAMBLING,
AND PABLO FERNANDEZ

Indigenous Australians are regarded as a priority in the Australian healthcare system due to their higher burden of disease and injury when compared with nonindigenous Australians. Most of the data regarding health and mental health issues in the indigenous population are collected by the Australian government and, to a lesser extent, through health research projects. While government collected data shows that indigenous people suffer from higher rates of nearly all forms of chronic health problems, there is limited data in relation to mental health rates. As a result, proxy measures have been used and generalized to the national level.[1-3]

Accordingly, older studies and surveys from 1997 to 2000 estimate that suicide rates; anxiety and depression; hospitalization rates for diagnosed mental disorders; emergency department attendances for mental health and substance misuse-related conditions; and contacts with public community health services are three times the nonindigenous rate. However these rates are thought to be underestimated, as many indigenous people do not access regular health services, or delay seeking help until problems are severe, particularly in remote and rural communities.

For example, according to a study in 2008, 16% of the total disease burden experienced by indigenous Australians and Torres Straight Island peoples was attributed to mental illness.[4] The prevalence of mental health issues within the indigenous community was highlighted in a recent study by Jorm and colleagues, which found that indigenous people were 2.7 times more likely to experience high or very high levels of psychological distress.[4] Similarly, studies from 2000 to the present suggest that indigenous adults had a higher prevalence rate of high and very high scores on measures of psychological distress, ranging from about 50% to three times higher on all measures when compared with nonindigenous adults.[5] Although there are no reliable statistics, the data suggest that indigenous youth are exposed to significant risk factors implicated in the development of mental health problems as well as a higher prevalence of behavior problems when compared with nonindigenous children.[6]

Hospitalization for mental health and behavior disorders of indigenous people was documented at 2.1 times the rate of nonindigenous people, with the rate of intentional self-harm also being reported at 2 times higher on average and 5.2 times higher for 25- to 40-year-olds.[7,8] Nationally, the rate of suicide for the indigenous population has risen from 5% of total Australian suicides in 1991 to 50% in 2010, despite only 3% of the Australian population identifying as indigenous.[9] In Western Australia's Kimberley region, the rate of indigenous suicide is 100 times the national average, with an indigenous suicide estimated to occur every week.[9] Similarly, the indigenous youth suicide rate among Northern Australian communities is claimed to be the highest in the world.[9]

Mental illness and the paucity of services available to indigenous people not only impact them individually but also impact their families and the community in general. For example, cultural stress and mental health disorders can lead to negative intracommunity dynamics known as "lateral violence," where increases in violence are observed within communities rather than toward socioeconomic adversaries.[10] This can have an impact on the social and emotional well-being of the community; undermining resilience and exposing community members to trauma and distress, which may result in further violence and substance abuse.[4,10]

A range of causative factors has been identified as potential underlying causes for the current service gap to indigenous populations. Social and cultural dislocation may be one factor that has resulted in high unemployment, fewer educational qualifications, lower income, adverse life events, smoking, and chronic physical illnesses. These related socioeconomic consequences are known as "mental health risk factors" and are experienced at significantly higher rates by indigenous people. Social disadvantage is also associated with behavior problems among children. While overcoming many of these problems requires a policy response from governments, it also requires targeted mental health intervention for individuals and families.[10-13]

Among other underlying causes, the barriers to accessing timely and appropriate health services have been identified as important reasons for the high level of unmet needs regarding mental health problems among indigenous Australians. The majority of indigenous Australians are known to be presently living in rural and remote areas where specialist healthcare services, including mental health services, are significantly lacking. The National Mental Health Commission has determined that the mental health services available to indigenous Australians are inadequate.[14] According to the 2011 Census, around two-thirds (65.2%) of indigenous Australians live outside of major metropolitan areas.[10] In the 2004–2005 National Aboriginal and Torres Strait Islander Health Survey, 15% of indigenous people were found to require a doctor in the previous 12 months but had not visited one, with cost determined to be one of the leading causes of avoiding health services.[10] Bailey (2005) has also suggested that a lack of education is another key barrier to avoiding health services.[15] Research has asserted that socioeconomic and racial factors serve as barriers to health services in indigenous people.[16]

TELEMENTAL HEALTH FOR INDIGENOUS AUSTRALIANS

There is evidence to suggest that telehealth can increase access to specialist mental health services[17,18] and, if used in suitable circumstances, may offer better patient outcomes.[19-21] Telemental health is one of the earliest branches of telemedicine, and also the first telemedicine activity recognized for Medicare reimbursement by the Australian government, as early as 2002. Since this time, there have been a large number of telemental health projects carried out in different parts of Australia, some of which have been successfully integrated into routine practice.[22] With the majority of indigenous people living in rural and remote areas of Australia, it is not surprising that there have been significant efforts to deploy telemental health services focusing on these communities. According to the Telehealth Assessment Report 2011, telemental health has been a major intervention tool used in almost all states in Australia to provide services to remote indigenous communities.[23] However, for various reasons, information relating to the involvement of indigenous Australian communities in telemental health projects and services is extremely limited. The only known survey that reported telemental health services specifically focusing on Australian indigenous communities was carried out in 2001.[24] This national survey reported that among the 25 telemental health services available in Australia at the time, only 7% of these services focused on working with Aboriginal or Torres Straight Islanders.[24] One reason for the paucity of research and information available in this area may relate to issues of cultural sensitivity with reporting on indigenous peoples' involvement in telemental health services. Nonetheless, telemental health projects and services have been widely considered as a promising means to support individuals living in rural and remote areas, particularly indigenous communities.

There have been a number of projects initiated by local governments or the federal government to provide telemental health services to Australian indigenous communities. Literature on telemental health services in Australia suggests that the South Australia Rural and Remote Mental Health Service (RRMHS), founded in 1996, is one of the busiest and most experienced services in the world.[25] While the service focuses on rural and remote communities in general, due to the high percentage of indigenous people living in these areas, the service has developed a significant focus on these communities. The RRMHS began to use videoconferencing from the outset to provide telemental health,[26] which subsequent studies showed was a safe and acceptable method of providing mental healthcare to indigenous communities.[27] As such, Alexander and Lattanzio have reported that a total of 271 consultations, over 2006 to 2009, were provided to rural and remote Aboriginal people living in South Australia.[25]

One important feature of the RRMHS has been the establishment of an Indigenous Mental Health Team with the aim of catering specifically to indigenous people. Team members are trained in the provision of telemental health services and are selected carefully to suit community needs with appropriate skills and qualities. This feature has been highlighted as a key factor for the success of this program.[25] The service has also served as a useful educational medium for health workers, with e-learning platforms such as video links being widely used to communicate within and outside the state to discuss matters relating to mental health issues affecting indigenous people.[28]

Another good example of telemental health service provision to indigenous communities can be found in Queensland, which has a large rural-based indigenous population. Using Queensland's extensive telehealth network, its public health department, Queensland Health, has been able to provide telemental health services to these communities. In practice, telemental health links are established between urban tertiary hospitals and rural and remote clinics to provide specialist mental health services along with other specialties. In addition, the Queensland Transcultural Mental Health Centre (QTMHC) has been a pioneer in using telehealth to provide services to communities. This statewide service provides information, referrals, and clinical consultations relating to mental health using a combination of face-to-face and videoconferencing consultations depending on an individual's ability to travel to a healthcare site. In some cases, face-to-face patient–clinician consultations are carried out using videoconferencing. In some other cases, videoconferencing is used for case conferences where a group of clinicians might discuss the patient's management plans.

Other Australian states have also increasingly made use of telemental health to provide services to rural and remote areas, including indigenous communities. According to the 2011 Telehealth Assessment Report, the Greater Southern Area Health Service (GSAHS) in New South Wales is using telehealth consultations provided by its Mental Health Emergency Care Support Centres (MHECS) to support an integrated model of mental healthcare for both acute and primary healthcare services. Clients of these services include a significant number of indigenous communities.[23] The Northern Territory, with its large indigenous population, has also been exploring ways and means to improve its mental health service. Herein, there have been a number of projects using telemental health applications, such as the Health-e-Towns project, of which indigenous communities are obvious beneficiaries.[23] A number of other Australian states, including Victoria, Western Australia, and Tasmania, have also piloted and implemented telemental health programs to rural and remote locations, however, to a lesser degree than those discussed.[24]

Evaluation of existing telehealth projects targeting indigenous communities has shown positive outcomes. For example, qualitative telehealth studies in oncology services for rural and remote North Queensland indigenous people were found to be appropriate with a high degree of user satisfaction from both mental health workers and the patients.[29] Likewise, published data from the Aboriginal Remote Telehealth (ART) project has reported positive results for the management of diabetes, renal disease, heart disease, and respiratory disease.[30] Indigenous peak health bodies (aboriginal representative bodies that seek to coordinate health services and matters related to health between the communities and the government) have also recognized the importance of telemental health as an important treatment medium, suggesting that the time is right for the increased rollout of telemental health services for indigenous peoples.[31] Evidence for the efficacy of telehealth services for indigenous Australians has important implications for the development of telemental health services to service these communities.

More broadly, extensive literature has shown that telemental health is a useful tool for providing services to indigenous communities.[31] Yet, even though literature relating to telemental health is becoming increasingly available, the evidence base for working with indigenous people is not strong. While few studies have evaluated telemental health projects in Australia, no known study has specifically examined aspects relating to the provision of mental health services to indigenous communities. In some cases, statistics on indigenous communities is not available, making it hard to assess the current status.[25]

Of the limited research available, several reviews have affirmed that the use of telemental health services with South Australian indigenous communities is feasible and beneficial to stakeholders.[24,32,33] Another study conducted in a New South Wales rural community used video-based telepsychiatric assessment to inform levels of patient risk and the need for transfer back to the regional center, and found that use of the technology did not alter the clinical judgment of the clinician regardless of the patient's Aboriginality. Furthermore, clinicians were found to be capable of making assessments that resulted in less acute risk being appropriately managed and a reduction in transfer rates back to the center. This study has important implications for telemental health technology and clinical practice in that assessing clinicians could potentially feel more confident in their assessment and that they have satisfied their ethical and medicolegal responsibilities to the patient.

BENEFITS TO THE INDIGENOUS

Telemental health services may reduce the unease indigenous people may feel when accessing nonindigenous mental health services by allowing culturally appropriate practitioners to provide services to a greater range of indigenous communities. Furthermore, indigenous health services may also provide a more culturally appropriate venue for attending telemental health sessions, as they are distributed across rural and remote areas as a result of specific government policy and funding. There is also the option for indigenous people to attend appointments remotely from a home computer; however, due to issues such as education, computer skills, access to suitable technology, and national bandwidth, further thought needs to be given to the types of telemental health interventions that may be considered suitable. For example, text-based telemental health services (e.g., self-help, e-mail–based or Web-chat-based therapy) may create challenges for indigenous people with lower levels of literacy, making visual-based talking sessions a better option. Opportunities also exist in the online environment to blend the technology interface to include visual screen tools, creative mediums, and other aids to assist with communication and treatment.[11] Telemental health services may also provide a more cost-effective method to reach indigenous people where economic issues restrict the availability of treatment services.[34] Such services offer mental health support through telephone, portable devices, and computer technologies to deliver a host of preventative and intervention services for a variety of psychological problems. Similarly, such services may also help overcome historical issues related to recruiting and retaining practitioners, due to a variety of factors including practitioner–environment fit, limited resources, and low support.[35] In view of the numerous barriers to service access and provision, the availability of telemental health may be of greatest benefit to rural and remote indigenous people. However, while research has shown the impact of telehealth in rural areas has generally been very positive on all measures examined,[12] it was not indigenous specific, and may have limited generality in drawing conclusions regarding impacts on indigenous populations.

BARRIERS AND POTENTIALS

Despite the widely acknowledged benefits that telemental health services are argued to be capable of providing to indigenous Australians, a number of barriers have been identified to effectively provide telemental health services to these communities. Firstly, there is a distinct lack of robust research evidence supporting its use with indigenous communities.[25]

Although there has been a significant increase in the popularity of tele-mental health service provision in Australia, accounting for at least one-third of all telehealth services in the country,[24] it remains a relatively understudied area of mental health service provision with insufficient data to draw formal conclusions regarding efficacy. The mixed nature of telemental health efficacy data may thus create further negative attitudinal barriers to service provision by mental health practitioners, particularly when coupled with relatively underdeveloped and uncertain safety, security, legal, and ethical safeguards that come with emerging technologies.[36] Furthermore, while the existing data is promising, there are various psychosocial, economic, and political risks in rolling out services to indigenous communities without understanding more about the best delivery methods, cultural appropriateness, and effectiveness of telemental health service provision for this population. It is unclear why there has been a lack of published research in this area. Even successful telemental projects have not published data on specific aspects of service delivery and outcomes in relation to indigenous service provision. It is unclear whether this is a result of evaluation design issues, capacity issues, or reluctance. In particular, while cultural appropriateness is widely acknowledged as being an important factor in the delivery of mental health services to indigenous people, it is still unknown which cultural issues act as barriers to providing telemental health care. This is a priority for research to elucidate how culturally sensitive issues or practices are best addressed so that telemental health services can be used in a culturally attractive and sensitive way for the benefit of these communities.[37]

Rural and remote areas where Australia's indigenous communities are based have a range of geographical and physical barriers to overcome. The availability of resources to such communities is another key barrier to telemental health, in that many indigenous people in rural and remote areas do not have access to the telephones, mobile devices, computers, the Internet, and videoconferencing technology that underpin these services. For example, so far, telemental health services to rural and remote areas have mainly concentrated on using videoconferencing technology. However, given that this technology often requires access to the high-quality equipment and communication infrastructure, there may be significant barriers to its optimal implementation and use.[27] Additionally, challenges exist in recruiting ongoing technicians for technology maintenance and staff training.[36] As such, it is important to explore other emerging technologies for the delivery of telemental health services. The use of Web-based technologies is one such approach that may be used in providing telemental health services to indigenous communities in Australia that makes use of less sophisticated and more widely accessible communication technology. For example, various studies have shown that Web-based technologies are useful for aiding with self-help and practitioner-guided treatments of mental illness.[38] Indeed, portable device technologies such as smartphones, tablets, and mobile apps are fast becoming accessible to all communities, with indigenous communities being no exception. In fact, at least one study has shown professional and community interest in developing mobile-based therapeutic applications for use by indigenous communities.[34] This is one of the first studies to explore the acceptability of e-mental health approaches for Aboriginal people among the health workforce. The outcome of the study may be an indication that as the use of mobile devices among the indigenous population expands, the opportunities for using such technologies to provide health services, including mental health services, may increase. Yet, in developing such services, it is important to integrate the social, emotional, cultural and spiritual values of the indigenous people to provide access to information about mental illness, local indigenous health services, online applications, and self-help tools to these communities.[39] The use of such technologies would further have to consider the literacy issues that often affect such communities and compensate for these by making use of simple language and highly visual- and/or audio-based modes of information and service provision. In addition, supporting government and nongovernment organizations such as Beyond Blue, Lifeline, Kids Helpline, Head Space, and National Aboriginal Community Controlled Health Organisation (NACCHO) to provide telemental health care to indigenous communities is an equally important endeavor given their existing branding, community connections, and communication technology infrastructure.

Lastly, similar to other fields of telemedicine, telemental health has still been constrained by a lack of appropriate medicolegal and ethical regulations. Indeed, many global ventures into telemental health practice have followed a model of assimilating what is done in face-to-face practice using distance modalities, without consideration of key issues such as professional regulation and licensure, variance in clinician–patient state laws, crisis management responses, informed consent, and confidentiality.[40] This is true for Australian practitioners too. It is vital that these obstacles be resolved before practitioners use telemental as a routine tool their clinical practice.

CONCLUSION

The importance of telemental health in improving mental health access for indigenous Australians living in small remote communities has been widely recognized. Accordingly, telemental health has been recognized as one of the key methods to closing disparities in health indices within this population. So far, it is anecdotally known that telemental health services may be a valuable tool for providing services to these communities; however, it is important to establish its efficacy through further research specifically focused on work with indigenous people. The conditions in which Australia's indigenous communities are presently living have also been equated with the developing world. If this is the case, then there is a rationale for exploring opportunities for using telemental health and telehealth in general, as it is often said that healthcare in the developing world is tightly linked with emerging technologies.

REFERENCES

1. Vos T, Barker B, Begg S, Stanley L, Lopez AD. Burden of disease and injury in Aboriginal and Torres Strait Islander peoples: the indigenous health gap. International Journal of Epidemiology. 2009;38(2):470–477.

2. Swan P, Raphael B. Ways forward: national Aboriginal and Torres Strait Islander mental health policy. Commonwealth of Australia 1995.

3. Vos DT, Barker B, Stanley L, Lopez A. The burden of disease and injury in Aboriginal and Torres Strait Islander peoples 2003. Centre for Burden of Disease and Cost-Effectiveness, School of Population Health, University of Queensland; 2007.

4. Jorm AF, Bourchier SJ, Cvetkovski S, Stewart G. Mental health of Indigenous Australians: a review of findings from community surveys. Medical Journal of Australia. 2012;196(2):118–121.

5. Australian Institute of Health and Welfare. Mental health services in Australia 2007–08. Canberra: AIWH, 2010. (AIWH Cat. NO. HSE 88; Mental Health Series No. 12).

6. Australian Indigenous HealthInfoNet. Social and emotional wellbeing (including mental health). http://www.healthinfonet.ecu.edu.au/. Accessed July 2015.

7. Holland C. Close the Gap-progress and priorities report The Close the Gap Campaign Steering Committee in February 2014. Paragon Printers Australasia. 2014.

8. Wilkes E, Gray D, Saggers S, Casey W, Stearne A. Substance misuse and mental health among Aboriginal Australians. Working Together. 2010:117.

9. McNamara PM. Adolescent suicide in Australia: rates, risk and resilience. Clinical Child Psychology and Psychiatry. 2013;18(3):351–369.

10. Australian Institute of Health and Welfare. Closing the Gap Clearinghouse: effective strategies to strengthen the mental health and wellbeing of Aboriginal and Torres Strait Islander People. 2014. https://www.google.com.au/webhp?sourceid=chrome-instant&ion=1&espv=2&ie=UTF-8#q=Australian+Institute+of+Health+and+Welfare.+Closing+the+Gap+Clearinghouse%3A+Effective+strategies+to+strengthen+the+mental+health+and+wellbeing+of+Aboriginal+and+Torres+Strait+Islander+People.+2014. Accessed July 2015.

11. Henderson S, Andrews G, Hall W. Australia's mental health: an overview of the general population survey. Australian and New Zealand Journal of Psychiatry. 2000;34(2):197–205.

12. Slade T, Johnston A, Oakley Browne MA, Andrews G, Whiteford H. 2007 National Survey of Mental Health and Wellbeing: methods and key findings. Australian and New Zealand Journal of Psychiatry. 2009;43(7):594–605.

13. Australian Bureau of Statistics. The health and wellfare of Australia's Aboriginal and Torres Strait Islander peoples. Canberra: ABS, 2010. (ABS Cat. No. 4704.4.0).

14. Australian Government National Mental Health Commission. A contributing life: the 2012 national report card on mental health and suicide prevention. Sydney: 2012.

15. Bailey J. You're Not Listening to Me!! Aboriginal mental health is different—don't you understand? Paper presented at 8th National Rural Health Conference 2005.

16. Otim ME, Kelaher M, Anderson IP, Doran CM. Priority setting in Indigenous health: assessing priority setting process and criteria that should guide the health system to improve Indigenous Australian health. International Journal for Equity in Health. 2014;13(1):45.

17. Brown FW. Rural telepsychiatry. Psychiatric Services. 1998;49(7):963–964.

18. Chung-Do J, Helm S, Fukuda M, Alicata D, Nishimura S, Else I. Rural mental health: implications for telepsychiatry in clinical service, workforce development, and organizational capacity. Telemedicine and e-Health. 2012;18(3):244–246.
19. Deslich SA, Thistlethwaite T, Coustasse A. Telepsychiatry in correctional facilities: using technology to improve access and decrease costs of mental health care in underserved populations. Permanente Journal. 2013;17(3):80.
20. Saurman E, Lyle D, Perkins D, Roberts R. Successful provision of emergency mental health care to rural and remote New South Wales: an evaluation of the Mental Health Emergency Care–Rural Access Program. Australian Health Review. 2014;38(1):58–64.
21. Roine R. The effectiveness of telemental health applications: a review. Canadian Journal of Psychiatry. 2008;53(11):769.
22. Simpson S, Reid C. Telepsychology in Australia: 2020 vision. Australian Journal of Rural Health. 2014;22(6):306–309.
23. Gray LC, Smith AC, Armfield NR, Croll P, Caffery LC. Brisbane: UniQuest University of Queensland. 2011. [2014-12-17]. webcite Telehealth Business Case, Advice and Options http://www.mbsonline.gov.au/internet/mbsonline/publishing.nsf/Content/E9F2448C7C016735CA257CD20004A3AE/$File/UniQuest%20Telehealth%20Business%20Case%20Advice%20and%20Options.pdf.
24. Lessing K, Blignault I. Mental health telemedicine programmes in Australia. J Telemed Telecare. 2001;7(6):317–323.
25. Alexander J, Lattanzio A. Utility of telepsychiatry for Aboriginal Australians. Australian and New Zealand Journal of Psychiatry. 2009;43(12):1185.
26. Yellowlees P, Kavanagh S. The use of telemedicine in mental health service provision. Australasian Psychiatry. 1994;2(6):268–270.
27. Fielke K, Cord-Udy N, Buckskin J, Lattanzio A. The development of an "Indigenous team" in a mainstream mental health service in South Australia. Australasian Psychiatry. 2009;17(Suppl 1):S75–S78.
28. Fielke K, Cord-Udy N, Buckskin J, Lattanzio A. The development of an "Indigenous team" in a mainstream mental health service in South Australia. Australasian Psychiatry. 2009;17(Suppl. 1):S75–S78.
29. Mooi JK, Whop LJ, Valery PC, Sabesan SS. Teleoncology for Indigenous patients: the responses of patients and health workers. Australian Journal of Rural Health. 2012;20(5):265–269.
30. Raven M, Butler C, Bywood P. Video-based telehealth in Australian primary health care: current use and future potential. Australian Journal of Primary Health. 2013;19(4):283–286.
31. Pilbeam, V., Ridoutt, L., Rich, J. and Perkins, D. (2014) Rural mental health service delivery models – a literature review, prepared for Mid North Coast Local Health District, Centre for Rural and Remote Mental Health.
32. Richardson LK, Christopher Frueh B, Grubaugh AL, Egede L, Elhai JD. Current directions in videoconferencing tele-mental health research. Clinical Psychology. 2009;16(3):323–338.
33. Monnier J, Knapp R, Frueh B. Recent Advances in Telepsychiatry: An Updated Review. Psychiatric Services. 2003;54(12):1604–1609. doi:10.1176/appi.ps.54.12.1604.

34. Dingwall KM, Puszka S, Sweet M, Nagel T. "Like Drawing into Sand": acceptability, feasibility, and appropriateness of a new e-mental health resource for service providers working with Aboriginal and Torres Strait Islander people. Australian Psychologist. 2015;50(1):60–69.

35. Conomos AM, Griffin B, Baunin N. Attracting psychologists to practice in rural Australia: the role of work values and perceptions of the rural work environment. Australian Journal of Rural Health. 2013;21(2):105–111.

36. Monthuy-Blanc J, Bouchard S, Maïano C, Séguin M. Factors influencing mental health providers' intention to use telepsychotherapy in First Nations communities. Transcultural Psychiatry. 2013;50(2):323–343.

37. Shore JH, Savin DM, Novins D,Manson SM. Cultural aspects of telepsychiatry. Journal of Telemedicine and Telecare. 2006;12(3):116–121.

38. Hickie HCIB. Using e-health applications to deliver new mental health services Medical Journal of Australia. 2010;192(11):53.

39. Mental Health First Aid. https://mhfa.com.au/. Accessed July 2015.

40. Childress CA. Ethical issues in providing online psychotherapeutic interventions. Journal of Medical Internet Research. 2000;2(1).

10

Refugee Telemental Health in Denmark

DAVOR MUCIC

Around the globe, ethnic and racial minorities experience a disproportionately higher burden from unmet mental health needs.[1-5]
Among ethnic and racial minorities, in comparison with the
majority group, mental illness may be even more stigmatized.[6]

The lack of a shared language between the healthcare professional and
the migrant is likely to be an obstacle to adequate healthcare delivery.
Language barriers are associated with lower rates of patient satisfaction
and poor care delivery in comparison with care received by patients who
speak the language of the care provider.[7-8]

Patients who face language barriers are less likely than others to have
a usual source of medical care; frequently receive preventive services at
reduced rates; have an increased risk of nonadherence to medications; are
less likely than others to return for follow-up appointments after visits to
the emergency room; and have higher rates of hospitalization and drug
complications.[9]

Several studies have found that language barriers are associated with lower rates of patient satisfaction and poor care delivery in comparison with care received by patients who speak the language of the care provider.[7-8]

The presence of a third person (i.e., an interpreter) in a confidential relationship affects patient satisfaction, as it influences both transference and countertransference between individuals involved, with unavoidable consequences on a doctor–patient relationship.[10]

Further, interpreter-mediated communication is linked to increased risk of loss of confidentiality, which is why most refugees, asylum seekers, and migrants exposed to such communication tend to be suspicious, wondering, "How soon will everyone in this little city speak about my illness?" Nevertheless, most ethnic minority migrants have brought their stigma already from their respective home countries.

Mistakes in interpretation (omissions, distorted questions, additions) occur frequently due to the common practice where family members and untrained interpreters serve as mediators in doctor–patient communication.[11-13] The use of a shared language (whether that of the patient or a third language shared by both patient and clinician) seems to be the most effective approach to ensure patient satisfaction and mutual comprehension.[14]

Common strategies for overcoming linguistic discordance and conducting reliable cross-cultural assessments are to use:

1. Professionally trained medical interpreters;
2. Ad hoc interpreters, for example, family members, friends, and bilingual clinicians of other specialties than the one patient refers to;
3. Culturally competent bilingual clinicians who have the same ethnic and cultural background as their respective patients (known as the "ethnic matching" model).

"Ethnic matching" appears to be the most desirable model used in addressing language barriers and cultural disparities in mental healthcare provision. Ethnic matching, supplemented by cultural competency training, has been proved as a common strategy to address a number of barriers in transcultural-related healthcare provision.[4,15]

However, the ethnic matching model is not that easy to implement. When the patient and the "matching" clinician are located in different places then a consultation is likely to require travel, either for the patient or the clinician. That is why telemental health (TMH) became an obvious solution and a basis for the telepsychiatry projects that are described in this chapter.

TELEPSYCHIATRY FOR REFUGEES AND ASYLEES IN DENMARK

Inadequate mental health services and mental health disparities for ethnic and racial minorities have been recognized in Denmark as well. A number of barriers to treatment have been observed and are related to well-known cultural and linguistic barriers as well as to limitations of the (mental) health system itself.

Effective interventions to address the previously mentioned challenges require innovation, the capacity to "think outside the box," cultural competence, and institutional support. The use of telecommunication technologies may provide innovative and effective means of responding to the needs of immigrant patients. A promising innovative model developed in early 2000 by Little Prince Treatment Centre in Copenhagen is described in this chapter. It relies on the use of videoconferencing in order to connect the patients with culturally competent bilingual clinicians without using interpreters.

While various telepsychiatry applications have been tested and developed over the last 5–6 decades, there are relatively few published reports describing the use of telepsychiatry in the provision of mental healthcare to cross-cultural patients.[16–19]

The first telepsychiatry pilot project in Denmark ever was conducted in August 2004. The aim of the project was to overcome the burden of poor service access for ethnic minorities in Denmark and promote a new way of delivering mental healthcare by use of videoconferencing in real time (aka synchronous telepsychiatry).[20] Thereafter, different approaches have been described dealing with specific needs of Hispanics/Latinos, Asians,[21-24] and Native Americans.[25,26]

The Little Prince Treatment Centre in Copenhagen has more cross-cultural expertise in telepsychiatry than other places in Europe.[27] The Centre is a private clinic that specializes in treating ethnic minorities, and its affiliated clinicians are bilingual, culturally competent mental health professionals. The hypothesis behind the project was that the majority of cross-cultural patients would prefer contact in their mother tongue, even if provided via telepsychiatry, rather than interpreter-provided face-to-face contact with a Danish doctor.

When the Centre launched the pioneer telepsychiatry pilot project in Denmark, ethnic minorities amounted to 8.2% of the country's population,[28] and mental healthcare was burdened by long waiting periods (3–6 months at private practitioners and even 12–36 months at specialized centres for treatment of refugees and torture victims); there was also a lack of bilingual resources, and most services were provided via interpreters. Four stations (i.e., two hospitals, one asylum seekers centre, and one social institution for rehabilitation of refugees and migrants) were connected via videoconference with the Little Prince Treatment Centre in Copenhagen. Bilingual clinicians affiliated with the Centre made it possible to assess and/or treat patients via their own language, to enhance reliable assessment, and to provide valid treatment for a wide variety of psychiatric disorders.

Several specialized centres for treatment of refugees and torture survivors were contacted and asked to participate in the project. They were offered technical support and necessary videoconferencing equipment without charge (market price about 10,000 €) in order to participate in the project where their patients could receive treatment by bilingual "ethnic" psychiatrists. A 9-item semistructured interview was designed in order to determine specialized centres clinicians' attitudes toward the project and telepsychiatry generally (Box 10.1). After 1–2 hours of information about telepsychiatry and about the project in Denmark, clinicians answered the semistructured interview.

Box 10.1   CLINICIANS' ATTITUDES TOWARD TELEPSYCHIATRY QUESTIONNAIRE

1. Do you think that the treatment of refugees/immigrants via translator is optimal?
2. Would you prefer to use ethnic clinicians rather than treatment via translators?
3. Do you have bad experiences with ethnic clinicians? If "yes," which?
4. What do you know about telepsychiatry?
5. What do you perceive are the advantages of telepsychiatry?
6. What do you perceive are disadvantages of telepsychiatry?
7. What are you most concerned about regarding potential participation in the project?
8. Do you perceive using translators as a better solution? If "yes," why ?
9. Have you ever asked your patients whether they would prefer an ethnic clinician rather than contact via translator?

Furthermore, a patient satisfaction questionnaire was designed (Table 10.1) for completion at the end of the visit. In this pilot phase, high acceptance and satisfaction were found regardless of the patients' ethnicity or educational level.[29] All patients preferred "remote" contact compared to in-person care with an interpreter, due to perceived higher anonymity, confidence/trust in providers, and self-efficacy to express intimate thoughts and feelings without a third person involved.[29] As expected, there was a clear correlation between the number of sessions, reported satisfaction level, and quality of care.[29] The patients' judgment of enhanced safety and comfort of TMH might also be due to less likelihood of meeting the doctor on the street and the risk of spreading rumors in the patients' neighborhood; this resembles the experience of Native American populations in small tribes in the United States.[30]

The telepsychiatry service continued after the pilot project ended in October 2007 and still operates regularly between a psychiatric office in Rønne (Bornholm Island) and Little Prince Treatment Centre in Copenhagen.

TABLE 10.1 USER SATISFACTION QUESTIONNAIRE

		Strongly Agree (%)	Agree (%)	Disagree (%)	Strongly Disagree (%)	Don't know (%)
1	I did get enough information about telepsychiatry					
2	I found the "encounter via TV" to be uncomfortable					
3	I did feel safe during telepsychiatry encounter					
4	I was satisfied with the sound quality					
5	I was satisfied with the picture quality					
6	I was able to achieve my goal via telepsychiatry/was able to express everything I wanted to					
7	I would recommend telepsychiatry to others					
8	I would prefer an encounter via an interpreter in the future					
9	What advantages did you perceive of telepsychiatry contact?					
10	What disadvantages did you perceive of telepsychiatry contact?					

Telepsychiatric assessments of hospitalized suicidal patients are particularly useful, especially when it comes to patients that have had a telepsychiatric contact prior to involuntary admission. Narratives from daily clinical work may significantly increase the understanding and acceptance of TMH among professionals with no TMH-related experience or professionals who are still in doubt, so I share the following story, which occurred during the first pilot project:

> NN, a 38-year-old male, refugee from Bosnia-Herzegovina, was diagnosed with PTSD and treated via telepsychiatry for 1 year prior to involuntary hospitalization. He was hospitalized due to increased suicide risk and suicidal threats. NN presented to his general practitioner, who decided to send him to the psychiatric emergency department located on the island where NN lives. There, NN was assessed by a Danish psychiatrist via a Bosnian interpreter and involuntarily hospitalized. A day later, NN was seen by the psychiatrist who had monthly encounters with him via telepsychiatry. It was very convenient for the psychiatric department located on an isolated island to call the psychiatrist who spoke the same language as the patient and who knew the patient best in order to assess the patient's mental state, including the current risk of suicide. Despite the fact that the consultation was done remotely, NN could disclose much more via TV using his native language than via interpreter under face-to-face consultation with the Danish doctor the day before. After the telepsychiatric consultation the patient remained on the ward for observation but was discharged the following day.

INTERNATIONAL TELEPSYCHIATRY

The most comprehensive international cross-border telepsychiatric service in the world was established in Denmark in mid-2006 (May 2006–October 2007) as a part of the cross-cultural telepsychiatric pilot project mentioned.[31] Because cross-cultural resources were more readily available in Sweden than in Denmark, it was desirable to involve cross-cultural clinicians from Sweden in the project. Furthermore, bilingual psychiatrists have not only the selected skills but also a detailed knowledge of the mental healthcare system in Scandinavia as well as knowledge about health systems in the patients' respective home countries. Videoconferencing equipment connected the Swedish office of the Little Prince Psychiatric Centre with the previously mentioned four stations during period of 18 months. Overall, high patient satisfaction was reported and minor disadvantages of telepsychiatry were offset by the fact that the doctor–patient language and cultural matching encouraged acceptance. The use of bilingual clinicians with similar ethnic and cultural backgrounds to their patients compensates for the distance and lack of physical presence.

The crucial indicators of patient satisfaction were:

- Accessibility of culturally competent care via the mother tongue;
- Ability to express intimate thoughts and feelings from a distance, without third-person involvement;
- Perceived safety and comfort of the service;
- High quality of sound and picture;
- Time savings associated with no need for travel;
- Reported willingness to use telepsychiatry again and recommending it to others;
- Preference for telepsychiatry in comparison to interpreter-assisted care.

Aside from projects developed by Little Prince Treatment Centre, a recently launched European project has potential to enhance the quality of care of ethnic minorities in the future. The MasterMind (**MA**nagement of MH di**S**orders **T**hrough advanc**E**d technology and se**R**vices—telehealth for the **MIND**) project was launched in March 2014 (ending in February 2017).[32] Relevant to this chapter is one of the project's three aims: "To explore the implementation of cultural and language specific computerized CBT services to EU citizens resident in another EU country i.e. online services in

Turkish for Turkish-speaking citizens in Denmark." Experiences gained from this project shall result in a set of guidelines, and a toolbox for the promotion and facilitation of implementation of a safe and effective e-mental health service across Europe.

DISCUSSION

Next we will discuss attitudes of both providers and patients towards the use of technological means in providing mental health services. Understanding these experiential attitudes has a great implication going forward when scaling up the applicability of TMH in various settings.

Professionals' Perspective

The impact of information on attitudes toward the use of technology in mental healthcare provision is not negligable,[33] as providers' attitudes toward telepsychiatry improves with "knowing" more about it. Commonly, professionals prioritize face-to-face contact with the patient, mentioning a number of potential obstacles that might occur during a videoconference ("What about body language," " I miss a smell," "What about Internet connection errors?" etc.). While there was general acceptance of telepsychiatry in our semistructured interview answered by the specialists employed in our projects who also have experience in treatment of refugees, we were surprised to see the lack of willingness to participate in the project as it was designed. Specialists did not assume the language was a crucial tool in psychotherapeutic work with ethnic minorities. They expressed reluctance toward the aim of the project and would prefer to use translators. Their argument was that "the language is not important but the competence of both translators and clinicians are of crucial importance." Some of specialists assumed their patients are "too ill to be involved in telepsychiatry contact." At the same time they expressed willingness to participate in the project by using the offered equipment "in order to reach as many patients as possible" (i.e., patients referred from remote areas) but not using the bilingual cross-cultural expertise from Little Prince Treatment Centre.[36]

The clinicians' attitudes and perceptions of TMH influence their intention to use the technology with their patients. However, the key predictor of the intention to use TMH is not clinicians' attitude toward it but essentially how useful they expect it to be for their cross-cultural patients. Perceived usefulness will have a positive impact on attitudes toward the technology, and perceived ease of use will positively influence perceived usefulness.[35] Findings suggest also that mental health workers have overall positive attitudes toward the use of TMH—particularly for clients in remote and rural locations,[35] which is in accordance with our experiences in Denmark.

Patients' Perspective

While patients entering mental health services usually have many concerns, those who were involved in TMH were largely accepting of it regardless of the type of service setting. Those who were asylum seekers wondered whether interpreters, depending on their nationality, would translate correctly (e.g., "One can never know whether they are translated correctly or not. That's why I prefer one that speaks my language." Or: "One can never trust them. Today I speak with the doctor and tomorrow the whole city knows everything about it." "They (Serbs/Albanians) have tortured me in Kosovo, so how can I trust them now?")[28]

Ethnicity did not appear to be associated with the patients' attitudes toward telepsychiatry. Differences in perception of the service were identified with respect to the patients' previous experiences with the mental health system in Denmark. Patients who had earlier received treatment via interpreters in Denmark were more favorable to telepsychiatry provided in the mother tongue, compared with patients without previous interpreter-related experiences. It was easier for the patients to express themselves from a distance, and they actually felt more secure and could control the situation, which resulted in them being more open. This goes against the general belief, where the lack of the direct face-to-face contact between patient and therapist in telepsychiatry often has been used as an argument against its use, even though international research shows that patient satisfaction is just as high and the treatment at least as effective via telepsychiatry as via conventional in-person contact.[36-38]

There is no doubt that some patients will prefer remote consultations due to the ability to control the presence of the psychotherapist so as to feel less influenced by him/her, that is, having the opportunity to "switch off" the therapist. In contrast, regarding countertransference issues, it has been noticed that some psychiatrists are reluctant to carry on mediated psychotherapy, which might deter the patients from asking or exploring for this possibility.[39]

It is possible, however, that some patients will have worries regarding security in connection with telepsychiatry sessions. However, the continuity maintained by seeing the same doctor no matter where the patient is located is probably one of the most important advantages of the described projects and services compared with traditional mental healthcare provision.

Of course, it is possible that some individuals will prefer communication via interpreter rather than via mother tongue, for example, torture victims who are suspicious and very much concerned about the doctor's ethnic origin, for example, Serbs versus Albanians (Serbia-Kosovo); Hutu versus Tutsi (Rwanda), and so on. Nevertheless public health should offer different options and let the patient choose voluntarily the one that is suitable for him/her in a specific situation. By increasing the range of patient choices we foster provider competition as well. Then we may speak about equal quality of care for all.

In a recent study the author suggests that increasing public awareness of the use and effectiveness of technology may help facilitate patients' acceptance.[39] However, when the only alternative to videoconference via respective mother tongue is mental healthcare provision via interpreters, then the patient's acceptance of remote consultation is expected. At the same time, overcoming cultural barriers requires strategies for training providers and increases their exposure to the TMH applications in order to increase their awareness of its applicability.

Finally, promising results of the international telepsychiatry project in Denmark, and cross-cultural telepsychiatry approach in general, might pave the way for potential development of an international telepsychiatry service where bilingual professionals all over the globe would be able to share their knowledge and expertise in order to assess and/or treat mentally ill ethnic minorities via their respective mother tongues. Clinical and scientific objectives and goals of such international TMH service as well as the potential outcomes of these are endless.[40]

CONCLUSION

As immigration is reality in almost every European country, it has become increasingly evident that standard treatment approaches require modification or adaptation in order to ensure that all patients receive effective mental healthcare. The use of TMH applications (videoconference, Web-based approaches and various e-mental–health apps) enables opportunities to build bridges over cultural and linguistic barriers by connecting patients with professionals that "match" culturally and linguistically. Within clinical practice, we have never been presented with a tool that requires so little investment in return for so much as is the case with TMH. Right now there is only one sustainable telepsychiatry service in Europe to treat ethnic minorities via TMH. After the pilot project ended in 2007, the service continued between a psychiatric practice on Bornholm Island and Little Prince Treatment Centre in Copenhagen. This is to our knowledge the only such service in the EU where assessment and treatment of ethnic minorities is provided via bilingual specialists through videoconferencing and mostly no use of interpreters.

When TMH becomes accepted as a supplemental tool to enhance quality of care and ease daily clinical work, then we will probably see the use of the technology on a larger scale. However, in the meantime healthcare providers have to understand the importance of communication processes to the healthcare encounter.

If problems mentioned are to be solved, significant changes to the mental health field must be made. One may hope that promotion and further development of TMH will lead to useful solutions capable of increasing the quality of care not only toward ethnic minorities but also toward the domestic Danish patient population.

REFERENCES

1. US Department of Health and Human Services. Mental health: culture, race, and ethnicity; a supplement to Mental health: a report of the surgeon general. Rockville, MD: US Department of Health and Human Services; 2001.
2. Alverson HS, Drake RE, Carpenter-Song EA, Chu E, Ritsema M, Smith B. Ethnocultural variations in mental illness discourse: some implications for building therapeutic alliances. Psychiatric Services. 2007;58:1541–1546.
3. Craig T, Jajua P, Warfa N. Mental healthcare needs of refugees. Psychiatry. 2006;5:405–408.
4. Ton H, Koike A, Hales RE, Johnson JA, Hilty DM. A qualitative needs assessment for development of a cultural consultation service. Transcultural Psychiatry. 2005;42:491–504.
5. Bhugra D. Migration and mental health. Acta Psychiatrica Scandinavica. 2004;109:243–258.
6. Leong FTL, Kalibatseva Z. Cross-cultural barriers to mental health services in the United States. Cerebrum. 2011;2011:5.
7. Carrasquillo O, Orav EJ, Brennan TA, Burstin HR. Impact of language barriers on patient satisfaction in an emergency department. Journal of General Internal Med. 1999;14:82–87.
8. Sarver J, Baker DW. Effect of language barriers on follow-up appointments after an emergency department visit. Journal of General Internal Medicine. 2000;15:256–264.
9. Flores G. Language barriers to health care in the United States. New England Journal of Medicine. 2006;355:229–231.
10. Spiegel JP. Cultural aspects of transference and countertransference revisited. Journal of American Academy of Psychoanalysis. 1976;4:447–467.
11. Brooks TR. Pitfalls in communication with Hispanic and African-American patients: do translators help or harm? Journal of NationalMedical Association. 1992;84(11):941.
12. Brua C. Role-blurring and ethical grey zones associated with lay interpreters: three case studies. Communication and Medicine. 2008;5(1):73.
13. Carlson J. Breaking down language barriers: hospital interpreters get credentialed with new certification programs. Modern Healthcare. 2010;40(46):32–34.

14. Riddick S. Improving access for limited English-speaking consumers: a review of strategies in health care settings. Journal of Health Care of the Poor and Underserved. 1998;9:40–61.

15. Jerrell JM. Effect of ethnic matching of young clients and mental health staff. Cultural Diversity and Mental Health. 1998;4:297–302.

16. Yellowlees PM, Odor A, Burke MM, et al. A feasibility study of asynchronous tele-psychiatry for psychiatric consultations. Psychiatric Services. 2010;61(8):838–840.

17. Sherrill WW, Crew L, Mayo RM, et al. Educational and health services innovation to improve care for rural Hispanic communities in the U.S. Education for Health (Abingdon). 2005;18:356–367.

18. Shore J, Kaufmann LJ, Brooks E, et al. Review of American Indian veteran telemental health. Journal of Telemedicine and e-Health. 2012;18(2):87–94.

19. Yeung A, et al. A study of the effectiveness of telepsychiatry-based culturally sensitive collaborative treatment of depressed Chinese Americans. BMC Psychiatry. 2011;11:154.

20. Mucic D. Telepsychiatry in Denmark: mental health care in rural and remote areas. Journal of eHealth Technology and Application. 2007;5(3).

21. Moreno FA, Chong J, Dumbauld J, et al. Use of standard webcam and Internet equipment for telepsychiatry treatment of depression among underserved Hispanics. Psychiatric Services. 2012;63(12):1213–1217.

22. Nieves JE, Stack KM. Hispanics and telepsychiatry. Psychiatric Services 2007;58(6):877.

23. Ye J, Shim R, Lukaszewski T, et al. Telepsychiatry services for Korean immigrants. Journal of Telemedicine and e-Health. 2012;18(10):797–802.

24. Chong J, Moreno F. Feasibility and acceptability of clinic-based telepsychiatry for low-income Hispanic primary care patients. Journal of Telemedicine and e-Health. 2012;18(4):297–304.

25. Shore JH, Brooks E, Savin D, Orton H, Grigsby J, Manson SM. Acceptability of telepsychiatry in American Indians. Journal of Telemedicine and e-Health. 2008;14(5):461–466.

26. Weiner MF, Rossetti HC, Harrah K. Videoconference diagnosis and management of Choctaw Indian dementia patients. Alzheimer's and Dementia 2011;7(6):562–566.

27. www.denlilleprins.org

28. Udlændingestyrelsen (Nøgletal på udlændingeområdet), 2004.

29. Mucic D. Transcultural telepsychiatry and its impact on patient satisfaction. Journal of Telemedicine and Telecare. 2010;16(5):237–242.

30. Hilty DM, Yellowlees PM, Tarui N, et al. Mental health services for California American Indians: usual service options and a description of telepsychiatric consultation to select sites. In: Ramesh M, Shahram K, eds. Telemedicine. Rijek, Croatia: InTech Open Press; 2013:75–104.

31. Mucic D. International telepsychiatry: a study of patient acceptability. Journal of Telemedicine and Telecare. 2008;14:241–243.

32. www.mastermind-project.eu

33. Casey LM, Joy A, Clough BA. The impact of information on attitudes toward e-mental health services. Cyberpsychology, Behavior, and Social Networking. 2013;16(8):593–598.

34. Mucic D. Telepsychiatry pilot-project in Denmark: videoconference by distance by ethnic specialists to immigrants/refugees. World Cultural Psychiatry Research Review. 2007:3–9.

35. Simms DC, Gibson K, O'Donnell S. To use or not to use: clinicians' perceptions of telemental health. Canadian Psychology. 2011;52(1):41–51. http://dx.doi.org/10.1037/a0022275.

36. Ruskin PE, Silver-Aylaian M, Kling AM, et al. Treatment outcomes in depression: comparison of remote treatment through telepsychiatry to in-person treatment. American Journal of Psychiatry. 2004;161:8.

37. O'Railly R, Bishop J, Maddox K, Hutchinson L, Fisman M, Takhar J. Is telepsyhiatry equivalent to face-to-face psychiatry? Results from a randomized controlled equivalence trial. Psychiatric Services. 2007;58:836–843.

38. Urness D, et al. Client acceptability and quality of life: telepsychiatry compared to in-person consultation. Journal of Telemedicine and Telecare. 2006;251–254.

39. Kaplan E. Psychotherapy by telephone, videotelephone and computer videoconferencing. Journal of Psychotherapy Practice and Research. 1997;6:227–237.

40. Mucic D, Hilty DM. e-Mental health. Chapter 12. Switzerland: Springer International; 2016. doi 10.1007/978-3-319-20852-7.

Telemental Health Delivery for Rural Native American Populations in the United States

SHAWN S. SIDHU, CHRIS FORE, JAY H. SHORE,
AND ERIN TANSEY

According to the US Census Bureau, "American Indian or Alaska Native (AI/AN) refers to a person having origins in any of the original peoples of North and South America and who maintain tribal affiliation or community attachment." As of 2010, there were 2,932,248 individuals who identified as solely Native American in the United States; this number rose to 5,220,579 when including those who identified as Native American while also belonging to another ethnic group.[1] As of January 2015 there were 566 individually recognized tribes across the United States.[2]

BURDEN OF MENTAL HEALTH ISSUES IN NATIVE AMERICANS

Native Americans are a resilient cultural group with a strong sense of community, family, heritage, and tradition.[3] This sense of belonging and connectedness can be a significant protective factor against morbidity and mortality caused by mental illness.[4] However, Native Americans have also had to endure volumes of intergenerational and historical trauma. This includes not only the ramifications of colonialism, such as death, disease, and loss of homeland, but also a loss of cultural identity and practices that resulted from the widespread forced Anglicization of Native youth in boarding schools in the early 20th century.[5-7]

The impact of this trauma along with extreme poverty[8] has contributed to the disparately high amounts of physical and mental health morbidity and mortality in Native Americans, even when compared with other minority groups.[9] With regard to mental health, this disparity appears to hold true. The prevalence rate of suicide in Native Americans is 1.5 times the national rate.[10] The rates of post-traumatic stress disorder, alcohol dependence, disruptive behavior disorders, and comorbidity of substance use and psychiatric disorders are disproportionately higher in Natives.[11,12]

GAP IN ACCESS TO MENTAL HEALTH SERVICES IN NATIVE AMERICANS

Despite the apparent need for mental and behavioral health services for Natives living in rural America, access remains limited.[13] Healthcare through the Indian Health Service is available in states across the country, and those with such services often have great difficulty with referring patients to specialists.[14] Poverty can be a very significant deterrent to access. Unemployment ranges from 13.5% to 16.2% with a median income of $19,865, resulting in 31.7% of Native American families living below poverty.[15] This translates to many Native families being unable to afford transportation, prescription costs, and the costs of specialized procedures.[14]

Given history and the resultant significant historical trauma, some Native Americans have a mistrust of the Western medical system and its institutions. Furthermore, there have been research abuses that have furthered the sense of mistrust, and some tribes continue to fight for ownership of their biological data collected through research.[16]

Many Native American communities have strong ties to alternative and traditional healing methods and highly value tribal independence, sovereignty, and privacy. A paternalistic, forceful, or dismissive approach by those in Western medicine could easily contribute to decreased use of services in Native communities. This highlights the need for providers of Western medicine in Native communities to approach patients with respect, open-mindedness, and a sense of collaboration.[17] To this point, Native American patients appear more comfortable sharing information about their traditional beliefs when providers are perceived as receptive and willing to initiate discussions around this topic.[18] There is evidence to suggest that improved cultural competency can actually improve racial and ethnic healthcare disparities.[19]

EVIDENCE SUPPORTING TELEMENTAL HEALTH SERVICES IN NATIVE AMERICAN COMMUNITIES

Here evidence is presented first on acceptability and next on efficacy of telemental health in Native communities.

Acceptability of Telemental Health in Native American Communities

One possible solution to the tremendous disparity in access to mental health services for Native communities is the use of telemental health services. The use of this modality addresses many of the aforementioned barriers to access. First, it saves time and money for all involved. A recent cost comparison study found that telemental health sessions saved $31.42 per session by reducing travel costs for physicians, and $195.18 per session by doing the same for patients.[20] While there is an initial investment required to purchase telehealth equipment, this cost is recuperated through the savings. Many Native communities have accesses to institutions that already have a telehealth infrastructure in place, such as the Indian Health Services, tribal health centers, local schools, or tribal colleges. Second, telemental health allows providers to live in urban areas while still providing care to rural and underserved communities, addressing rural recruitment and retention issues. A survey following trainees from the University of New Mexico Rural Psychiatry Residency Program found that while 95% of respondents continued to work with rural and underserved populations, only 26% reported living in the communities they treated.[21] The most commonly cited reasons for this were professional isolation, long travel distances, and limited educational opportunities for children. Telemental health allows such providers to continue practicing rural medicine while meeting other family obligations and needs. Third, increasing the number of available providers for rural communities would lead to decreased wait times between appointments, resulting in improved care and outcomes. Lastly, this would decrease the burden on other social agencies and institutions within the region that had been absorbing the impact of untreated mental illness (e.g., social services, juvenile and adult correctional services, emergency departments, etc.).

While there may be many compelling reasons to institute telemental health services in rural Native communities, none would be of any significance if Native American patients viewed this unconventional form of treatment unfavorably. While data on this topic is very limited, one study of Northern Plains American Indian male Vietnam veterans demonstrated that 94% of those surveyed had a general positive response to telemental health and 92% indicated a desire to use the service again.[22] Another study of three Northern Plains Veterans Administration clinics showed that while prior to implementation of telemental health services 67% of clinic staff participants reported a positive initial impression of telemental health and 10% reported mixed impression, after implementation of telemental health services 82% reported a positive impression and only 3% reported a mixed impression.[23]

A review of cultural aspects of telemental health[24] described several important considerations in providing culturally appropriate care that would likely increase American Indians acceptance of this form of healthcare delivery. First, programs build patient trust by employing a tribal/ telehealth outreach worker (TOW). This person was often a known and respected community member who would help with administrative duties and serve as a liaison with the tribal community and guide the treating psychiatrist in learning about cultural or local issues relevant to patient care. Second, the study authors recommended understanding patients' previous experiences with other healthcare organizations. In doing so, clinicians could better understand how the patients' acceptance (systems transference) might help or hinder their care. Third, they recommended educating all patients on confidentiality and being particularly sensitive to concerns of confidentiality for patients with psychotic disorders. Finally, in an effort to foster understanding, interest, and commitment to patients they suggested that periodic in-person visits might help facilitate a therapeutic relationship. [25]

Effectiveness of Telemental Health in Native American Communities

If telemental health is an acceptable form of treatment for some Native Americans, the next question is whether or not it is effective for treating mental health conditions in this group. There are several ways in which effectiveness can be measured.

One such way would be to compare the reliability of telemental health diagnoses as compared with in-person treatment. A 2007 study of 54 Northern Plains male veterans attempted to look at the reliability of using a diagnostic instrument (SCID, or Structured Clinical Interview for DSM) to make a psychiatric diagnosis in person compared with videoconferencing. For several major mood disorders (major depressive disorder, dysthymia, generalized anxiety disorder, panic disorder), assessments did not significantly differ between the two.[26] A notable limitation is the small study sample size.

Similarly, several studies in the United States in non-Native populations have shown telemental health can provide a reliable diagnosis of common psychiatric symptoms but more subtle signs such as emotional affect are less reliably assessed. This is particularly problematic for bandwidths lower than 128 kilobits per second (Kbps).[27] Currently, typical telemental health systems transmit at bandwidths between 128 and 512 Kbps.[28]

Another way to measure effectiveness would be to create a randomized controlled trial comparing telemental health with in-person treatment as they relate to outcomes. Unfortunately no such trials have been conducted in Native American populations to date. One RCT published in 2007[27] compared psychiatric treatment of telemental health to in-person treatment for 495 adult patients in Ontario, Canada. This study did not identify race or ethnicity of its participants; however, in a 2006 Canadian Census 8% of the city's total population was reported to be North American Indian.[29] The treatment model was a psychiatrist providing consultation and short-term follow-up to patients referred by their primary care providers for a wide range of psychiatric conditions in this rural, remote location. The services provided (medication recommendations, therapy referrals, and social service referrals) were found to be similar. They also noted the cost to deliver the care via technology was 10% less per patient than in-person service. Noted limitations included inability to detect subtle differences in clinical care and high study noncompletion rate of scales administered at 4-month follow-up.

A second randomized controlled trial examined children from underserved communities in the Pacific Northwest and found that telemental health services to treat ADHD performed better than a treatment model consisting of one telemental health consultation to the child's primary care provider.[30] The experimental telemental health service model in this study provided six sessions with combined medication management and caregiver behavioral training. The children were ages 5–12 years, and their ethnic/racial makeup was primarily European/White ancestry, so it is difficult to generalize these study results.

Lastly, a comprehensive literature review of 15 articles written between 2003 and 2013 by Hilty et al.[31] concludes that telemental health is effective for both diagnosis and assessment purposes across a multitude of populations including adults, children, geriatric patients, and ethnic groups. In addition, they found that telemental health appears to be comparable to in-person care and can be provided across a broad spectrum of medical settings, including emergency rooms and home health.

A DESCRIPTION OF CURRENT NATIVE AMERICAN
TELEHEALTH PROGRAMS IN EXISTENCE

A concrete programmatic description of two telemental health models is provided here for the purposes of illustrating how such programs are structured and the resources that are required.

University of Colorado Centers for AI/IN Health/Department of Veterans Affairs

Since 2001, collaboration within the Department of Veterans Affairs (VA), in partnership with the University of Colorado Centers for American Indian and Alaska Native Health (CAIANH), designed, implemented, and administered a unique program of telemental health clinics for American Indian veterans with post-traumatic stress disorder (PTSD). The VA is the large federal body in the United States that has been tasked with providing healthcare services to veterans. This includes an extensive network of inpatient hospitals, outpatient clinics, and even telehealth services. The clinics began in response to the identified needs of American Indian veterans and use a service delivery model that (1) provides ongoing mental healthcare such as medication management, case management, and individual, group, and family therapy; (2) uses Native American veteran volunteers to serve as outreach workers on-site and in the community (the Tribal Veterans Representative program);[32] (3) coordinates important community resources into care such as local traditional healers and/or the Indian Health Service.[24]

The ongoing development, implementation, and expansion of these clinics has been part of a program improvement process that has been well documented in a series of published articles, including controlled studies, program and case reports, and model descriptions.[24] This ongoing development effort has led to the expansion of the core of these clinics based out of Denver as well as a number of clinics based on this model. To date there have been 14 clinic sites working with over 20 different tribes. A 10-year review of activity (2002–2011) of the Denver-based clinics showed 970 clinic days held, 3,220 individual sessions, 440 groups, and a total of more than 4,600 patient contacts.[24] A number of evaluations have demonstrated the impact of this model in terms of potential for costs savings, and increasing access to and quality of care. The intersection of the university, VA, Indian Health Service, and tribal partners has brought a mix of resources and collaboration that has aided in the success of these clinics to date. No single organization has contained all the resources, knowledge, or infrastructure to allow a program like this to exist independently.

The Indian Health Service Telebehavioral Center of Excellence

The Indian Health Service Telebehavioral Health Center of Excellence (TBHCE) was established in 2008 and initially funded via the Methamphetamine and Suicide Prevention Initiative. The center's program was established to investigate the feasibility of providing telemental healthcare in Native communities. The Indian Health Service, not unlike the VA, is the large federal body tasked with providing healthcare to Native American populations throughout the country. The Indian Health Service too includes an extensive network of inpatient hospitals, outpatient clinics, and telehealth services, and is present in both rural and urban settings. Patients do need to have a proof of Native American status in the form of a Certificate of Indian Blood, for example, to receive services through the Indian Health Service. Care through the Indian Health Service, much like that through the VA, is largely free of cost to those who qualify, but does have some limitations with regard to medication formularies and specific treatments offered. The US Congress passed the Indian Self-Determination and Education Assistance Act in the 1970s, otherwise known as Public Law 93-638, which allowed the transfer of federal programming from large institutions such as the Indian Health Service back to tribes.[33] Therefore, while many Native American tribes across the United States today do receive medical services through the Indian Health Service, many also arrange for such healthcare services independently by contracting for and providing their own healthcare services with the same financial stream that would have funded the Indian Health Service.

Within the Indian Health Service, it was recognized that the traditional model of recruiting and retaining behavioral health providers in every community where they are needed was not viable for many of the reasons mentioned. The initial pilot was restricted to New Mexico, but quickly grew. This rapid growth indicated that telemental health is a viable option to meet the needs of many tribal communities and that it is an acceptable form of care. In fact, the Indian Health Service no longer differentiates telemental health from in-person mental healthcare, requiring a separate patient consent.

Initially the center's exclusive mission was to provide clinical care for mental health issues, with a particular focus on child and adolescent psychiatry, given the marked lack of services felt acutely across many rural Native communities. As the TBHCE has grown, mental health services have expanded to include, adult, addiction, geriatric, and infant mental health. Furthermore, in response to needs of our sites, the TBHCE now offers adult, child, and family therapy.

A second mission of the TBHCE, which has evolved in addition to expanding clinical services, is the creation of Web-based educational content for primary care and midlevel providers working in rural communities. Many Indian Health Service and tribal providers are located in frontier and rural areas, where obtaining the license-required continuing education (CE) credits is difficult. Thus the TBHCE has created a series of webinars in which content experts deliver interactive evidence-based lectures to the virtual audience. The webinars can be viewed in real time, downloaded, or streamed for viewing at a later time, and PowerPoint presentations are also made available for download. Webinars are delivered using Adobe Connect software, which includes the ability for participants to engage in a discussion with the presenter using chat windows, and also allows for the embedding of multiple-choice questions, which have now become a standard feature of every presentation.

Both missions of the TBHCE have met with success, and a third element of direct consultation to rural sites was also added. In Fiscal Year

2014, the TBHCE provided free training to more than 9,000 providers and awarded more than 5,000 continuing education credits. In the same period, TBHCE providers saw more than 2,800 patients via televideo. Most of these patients would have gone without care, were it not for these telemental health services. The center is currently providing care to 18 rural Native American communities across six states mostly clustered in the Mountain West but also on the East Coast. Currently there are a total of eight psychiatrists on staff, four of whom are also child psychiatry trained and one of whom is addiction psychiatry trained. The child psychiatrists on staff typically do see adults also depending on the need of each individual clinical site. The majority of psychiatrists on staff are only part-time, ranging anywhere from 10% to 50% of a full-time equivalent. There are currently therapists on staff as well, both a psychologist and a masters-level social worker.

IMPLEMENTATION OF TELEMENTAL HEALTH IN NATIVE AMERICAN POPULATIONS: BARRIERS, FACILITATORS, AND IMPROVEMENT FOR THE FUTURE

Here both barriers and facilitators to providing telemental health services in Native communities are discussed initially prior to assessing needed improvements and future directions.

BARRIERS

While telemental health has been a success in the programs described, it does carry with it some challenges. Transportation continues to be an issue for a significant portion of the population, as patients still have to travel from their home to the telehealth connection site (i.e., tribal health center or Indian Health Service clinic). For families without working vehicles, this poses the challenge of having to ask others for rides, arrange for Medicare/Medicaid pick-up, or find suitable public transportation. This is a challenge that will likely continue into the foreseeable future, or at least until technology becomes so cheap and readily available that patients will be able to connect from home. Even for institutions with special transportation programs, some patients may have to travel significant distances to get to the telehealth clinic. For communities in which there is not already an established telehealth connection site such as a clinic, hospital, or school, there is also the issue of an upfront cost investment. This could disproportionately affect tribes who are in charge of providing their own healthcare and do not have a contract with Indian Health Service or other healthcare agencies. Even if such tribes were to cover the upfront costs, there may be a lack of experience with this technology and limited technical support on their side. The quality of telemental health services provided, including audiovisual clarity, connection speed, and strength of connection continue to be an ongoing issue for even well-funded and heavily equipped institutions and agencies. Some regions of the country are so remote that the required bandwidth is simply not available regardless of the cost.

Although telemental health provides many conveniences to providers that were previously unavailable, some providers may continue to prefer to deliver care in a traditional face-to-face model. Some providers may shy away from temporary contracts with tribes, agencies, and/or institutions, and may be seeking employment opportunities where more benefits are offered. While telemental health may allow for a redistribution of mental health workers, it does little to address the core issue of a massive overall workforce shortage in mental health. Also, insurance reimbursement from both public and private entities is often out of date and providers may be unable to adequately bill for services.[14] This all being said, the data overwhelmingly suggests that those providers who do provide telemental health services are satisfied with their work.[22]

There are also several regulatory issues at play when it comes to telemental health. First is the issue of licensure. Providers must have a state medical license for each state in which they practice. Therefore, providing telemental health services across state lines would necessitate that the telemental health provider obtain a medical license for the state in which care is being provided. Federal entities such as the Indian Health Services and VA have the ability to bypass this requirement. Second, credentialing and malpractice can be very complicated, as the precedent set for both of these is in traditional medical environments. Access to providers over telemental health during nonworking hours may be more difficult, making the assessment of side effects and acute crisis management more difficult. These situations could theoretically result in malpractice claims, but could also be avoided with the proper protections, action plans, and access in place. Jurisdictional issues can be complicated as well, with states having vastly different laws on issues like civil commitment, police involvement with mental health, and minor age requirements to make medical decisions, to name a few.[34]

Lastly, perhaps one of the greatest barriers to telemental health in Native American populations could be the potential cultural divide between providers and patients. This requires that providers be sensitive to not only the cultural needs of their patients but also cultural norms with the clinic staff, families of patients, and other providers in the community. Yellowlees et al.[35] suggest that rural populations may have a greater degree of geographical isolation and unique cultural factors, including language, customs, and societal norms. They also point out that some rural areas may have a significantly higher rate of poverty and larger concentrations of ethnic populations. If not taken into account in a culturally sensitive way by the provider and the provider's institution, this could certainly pose a barrier to treatment. Shore et al.[25] suggest that providers consider the degree to which the patient's cultural identity and background influences their comfort around telemental health, and how differences between the patient and provider may influence this relationship. They go further to suggest that the more familiar providers are with the community of their patients, including frequent contact and open channels for feedback, the lesser the likelihood that cultural differences will become a complete barrier to treatment.

FACILITATORS

There are some facilitators that may help to offset some of the barriers to telemental health in Native American communities discussed. For communities in which there is existing infrastructure in place through other institutions and/or agencies connected to the tribe, there may be a way to offset upfront costs, and the technology required may already be available. Technical support and equipment upkeep may also be available through these sources. Telemental health may be seen by some third parties as an investment worth making. This may include anything from lobbying a local insurance company into starting up services in a particular area to applying for local and national service or research grants to start such services. Telemental health equipment in such communities can be used not only for patient care but also as a vehicle to deliver education and trainings to midlevel providers and other professionals in the community. This is already being done as part of the Indian Health Service TBHCE in partnership with the University of New Mexico and several other community partners, with multiple webinars being broadcast every month on a broad range of topics. This equipment is also used for case consultation and supervision services across great distances. The use of TOWs and Tribal Veterans Representatives previously described[24] is an example of how to make telemental health services more culturally adaptive and relevant, helping to address the issue of cultural barriers. Lastly, even given the limitations discussed, telemental health may be the only way to provide some populations with any care whatsoever. In this light, the tremendous need for services and the healthcare disparity that exists in many rural Native American communities is a facilitator in and of itself.

Improvements and Future Directions

Telemental health is a rapidly emerging treatment modality with considerable potential in rural Native American communities. Despite a seemingly exponential increase in interest over the past several decades, the field itself remains in its infancy. As mentioned, literature in many areas remains sparse. The next steps for proponents of this technology are to address current limitations and barriers while simultaneously continuing to develop smarter and more sustainable systems for the future.

In addition to improving the quality and availability of technology, those providing telehealth can continue to do an even better job reaching out to Native American communities around issues of perception and satisfaction. This collaboration could include anything from quality improvement measures to regular meetings with tribal elders and officials to address concerns. In such meetings, an open-minded and culturally sensitive approach would more likely result in a strong collaboration. This process also includes reaching out to on-site staff and other community providers including primary care physicians, nurses, social workers, other mental health providers, teachers, and any other involved parties. For example, the San Carlos Apache Wellness Center in Arizona reported initial difficulty in getting their local hospital and pharmacy to partner with a non–Indian Health Service psychiatrist to provide telehealth services. However, they were able to resolve this challenge by bringing the psychiatrist in to meet the hospital staff and getting the provider hospital credentialing and privileging. The Wellness Center partnered with several regional Arizona organizations and the Indian Health Service. In doing so, the San Carlos Apache mental health center was able to successfully establish a telemental health service that increased access to mental health services for 14,500 tribal members by six times more hours per month.[36]

Future directions also include ensuring that telemental health in Native communities is an investment that is viewed as financially sustainable. Some states such as Alaska have worked hard with lawmakers to craft progressive legislation improving Medicaid compensation schemes for medical care provided via video teleconferencing and telehealth. Alaska's telehealth services are also supported by more than 30 smaller organizations in addition to Medicaid.[14] This could prove to be an incredibly valuable strategy. First, states may be leery of investing in telehealth initially without any demonstrable outcome data. Therefore, states, agencies, and institutions who are just starting telehealth services may need to lean on smaller organizations or grants for funding. Targets for such grants might include local, patient-centered, and community-based participatory research funding sources in addition to traditional sources such as the Substance Abuse Mental Health Services Administration (SAMHSA) and the National Institutes of Mental Health (NIMH). Second, by building such an extensive network of support from smaller and midlevel organizations, the fate of telehealth does not rest in the hands of the annual state budget. Lastly, the approach of building support through smaller organizations also likely results in greater teamwork, rapport building, and community engagement as participants on both sides would need to work more closely with one another.

Another future direction would be to use the advancement of technology to help further the possibilities of telemental healthcare. This could include anything from improving connection quality to larger projects such as crafting comprehensive electronic medical record systems and networks. Such networks would allow for greater individual care as providers would have enhanced communication and the ability to follow a common treatment plan. The databases generated by these systems could also potentially allow for population-wide data analysis and quality improvement studies, not to mention valuable healthcare outcome data that could be shared with legislators, tribal members, or other interested parties. In outcome-based medical models such as that forecasted by the Affordable Care Act, the demonstration of improved care health outcomes with simultaneous decreases in cost is considered a gold standard and would be incredibly valuable for agencies providing telemental health services.[37] It should be noted that the upfront cost required for such systems might be more than many Native communities would be able to overcome; however, the creation of a unified electronic health record in large systems such as the VA and Indian Health Service might make this more of a possibility for tribes. While such institutions do technically have a comprehensive system, accessing information from another clinical site within the institution can be difficult and requires a series of complex steps, and the actual electronic medical record itself can vary from site to site. There would undoubtedly be costs to such large federal institutions to unify their medical records, but a cost analysis might demonstrate ways for the larger system to save valuable resources such as time and money by being able to track patients across multiple sites and systems.

Another potential application of technology would be to use mobile platforms to improve the access to care and the quality of care delivered. These applications could be geared toward providers, enabling greater remote access to patient data and the ability to perform actions such as prescribing medications or ordering labs from afar. These applications could also work to synthesize electronic medical records to create comprehensive patient profiles, including built-in quality improvement measures to reduce errors and customized reminders for providers. On the patient side such applications might allow for patients to remotely access their own health information; schedule appointments with greater ease, thereby increasing access; and receive reminders to maintain a healthy lifestyle and remain adherent to their individual medical treatment plans. Though many tribal communities have extremely limited or no mobile connectivity, in the not-too-distant future patients will connect through mobile applications from home for telemental health sessions. While such technological advances are certainly not limited to telemental health and would require significant efforts in patient education toward technological literacy, the access to technology that telemental health provides would lend itself very well to such advances.

CONCLUSION

In summation, despite suffering huge health disparities, Native Americans are a resilient and pragmatic people. Telemental health is a viable treatment model for delivering quality mental healthcare to Native American communities where the burden of mental health conditions and difficulty accessing care continue. There is evidence to suggest that Native American groups find telemental health to be an acceptable form of treatment with good efficacy. While many barriers to the use of telemental health in Native communities exist, there are simultaneously many facilitators of this treatment model. Future directions include addressing these barriers, improving collaboration with Native communities, ensuring telemental health remains financially viable, and using technology to expand the reach of this treatment modality.

NOTE

Disclaimer: The authors of this chapter are not in any way implying that all Native Americans are similar. Indeed, there are likely great differences on both a tribal and individual level that are not clearly expressed in this chapter. The data presented are general data collected from large numbers of Native Americans, but are far from representative of all Native Americans. Also, the views expressed in this article are those of the authors and do not reflect the position or policy of the Department of Veterans Affairs, Indian Health Services, or any of the other affiliated universities or institutions.

REFERENCES

1. Norris T, Vines PL, Hoeffel EM. The American Indian and Alaska Native Population: 2010 Census Briefs. US Census Bureau. Document Number C2010BR-10. 2012; 2. http://www.census.gov/prod/cen2010/briefs/c2010br-10.pdf. Accessed December 17, 2015.
2. Department of the Interior: Bureau of Indian Affairs. Indian entities recognized and eligible to receive services from the United States Bureau of Indian Affairs. Federal Register. 2015;80(9):1942–1948.
3. Mackin J, Perkins T, Furrer C. The power of protection: a population-based comparison of native and non-native youth suicide attempters. American Indian Alaska Native Mental Health Research. 2012;19(2):20–54.
4. Hill DL. Relationship between sense of belonging as connectedness and suicide in American Indians. Archives of Psychiatric Nursing. 2009;23(1):65–74.
5. Smith A. Soul wound: the legacy of Native American Schools. Amnesty International. March 26, 2007. Accessed December 17, 2015. http://www.amnesty-usa.org/node/87342
6. Child BJ. Boarding schools. In: Hoxie FE, ed. Encyclopedia of North American Indians: Native American history, culture, and life from Paleo-Indians to the present. 1996:80. Boston: Houghton Mifflin Harcourt.
7. Strickland C, Walsh E, Cooper M. Healing fractured families: parents' and elders' perspectives on the impact of colonization and youth suicide prevention in a Pacific Northwest American Indian tribe. Journal of Transcultural Nursing. 2006;17(1):5–12.
8. Krogstad JM. 1-in-4 Native Americans and Alaska natives are living in poverty. Pew Research Center. June 3, 2014. http://www.pewresearch.org/fact-tank/2014/06/13/1-in-4-native-americans-and-alaska-natives-are-living-in-poverty/. Accessed April 22, 2015.

9. Liao Y, Tucker P, Giles WH. Health status of American Indians compared with other racial/ethnic minority populations—selected states, 2001–2002. Morbidity and Mortality Weekly Report. 2003;52(47):1148–1152.

10. US Department of Health and Human Services. Mental health: culture, race, and ethnicity, a supplement to Mental Health: A Report of the Surgeon General. DHHS Publication Number 0-16-050892-4.Washington, DC: US Government Printing Office; 2001.

11. Beals J, Novins DK, Whitesell NR, et al. Prevalence of mental disorders and utilization of mental health services in two American Indian reservation populations: mental health disparities in a national context. American Journal of Psychiatry. 2005;162(9):1723–1732.

12. Beals J, Piasecki J, Nelson S, et al. Psychiatric disorders among American Indian Adolescents: prevalence in northern plains youth. Journal of the American Academy of Child and Adolescent Psychiatry. 1997;36(9):1252–1259.

13. Human J, Wasern C. Rural mental health in America. American Psychologist. 1991;46(3):232–239.

14. Hays H, Carroll M, Ferguson S, et al. The success of telehealth care in the Indian Health Service. American Medical Association Journal of Ethics. 2014;16(12):986–996.

15. US Department of Health and Human Services. Trends in Indian health. Public Health Service, Indian Health Service. Washington, DC: US Government Printing; 1994.

16. Harmon A. Indian tribe wins fight to limit research of its DNA. New York Times. April 21, 2010. http://www.nytimes.com/2010/04/22/us/22dna.html?pagewanted=all&_r=0. Accessed June 9, 2015.

17. Eggertson L. Doctors should collaborate with traditional healers. Canadian Medical Association Journal. 2015;187(5):E153–E154.

18. Shelley B, Sussman A, Williams R, et al. "They don't ask me so i don't tell them": patient-clinician communication about traditional, complementary, and alternative medicine. Annals of Family Medicine. 2009;7(2):139–147.

19. Brach C, Fraserirector I. Can cultural competency reduce racial and ethnic health disparities? a review and conceptual model. Medical Care Research and Review. 2000;57(1):181–217.

20. Horn BP, Barragan GN, Fore C, Bonham CA. A cost comparison of travel models and behavioural telemedicine for rural, Native American populations in New Mexico. Journal of Telemedicine and Telecare. 2015 May. Epub ahead of print. doi: 10.1177/1357633X15587171.

21. Bonham C, Salvador M, Altschul D, Silverblatt H. Training psychiatrists for rural practice: a 20-year follow up. academic psychiatry. 2014;38(5):623–626.

22. Shore J, Brooks E, Savin D, et al. Acceptability of telemental health in American Indians. Telemedicine and e-Health. 2008;14(5)461–466.

23. Brooks E, Spero M, Bair B. The diffusion of telehealth in rural American Indian communities: a retrospective survey of key stakeholders. Telemedicine and e-Health. 2012;18:60–66.

24. Shore J, Brooks E, Dialey N, et al. Review of American Indian veteran telemental health. Telemedicine and e-Health. 2012;18(2):87–94.
25. Shore J, Savin D, Novins D. Cultural aspects of telemental health. Journal of Telemedicine and Telecare. 2006;12:166–121.
26. Shore J, Savin D, Orton H. Diagnostic reliability of telemental health in American Indian veterans. American Journal of Psychiatry. 2007;164:115–118.
27. O'Reilly R, Bishop J, Maddox K. Is telemental health equivalent to face-to-face psychiatry? results from a randomized controlled equivalence trial. Psychiatric Services. 2007;58(6):836–843.
28. Deslich S, Stec B, Tomblin S. Telemental health in the 21st century: transforming healthcare with technology. Perspectives in Health Information Management. 2013;10:1f.
29. Germain, Marie-France. 2006 Aboriginal population profile for Thunder Bay. Statistics Canada. Government of Canada. http://www.statcan.gc.ca/pub/89-638-x/2009001/article/10832-eng.htm. Published January 29, 2010. Accessed July 1, 2015.
30. Meyers K, Vander Stoep A, Zhou C. Effectiveness of a telehealth service delivery model for treating attention-deficit/hyperactivity disorder: a community-based randomized controlled trial. Journal of the American Academy of Child and Adolescent Psychiatry. 2015;54(4):263–274.
31. Hilty DM, Ferrer DC, Parish MB, et al. The effectiveness of telemental health: a 2013 review. Telemedicine Journal and E-Health. 2013;19(6):444–454.
32. Kaufmann LJ, Buck Richardson WJ Jr, Floyd J, et al. Tribal Veterans Representative (TVR) training program: the effect of community outreach workers on American Indian and Alaska Native Veterans access to and utilization of the Veterans Health Administration. Journal of Community Health. 2014;39(5):990–996.
33. US Department of the Interior: Office of the Special Trustee for Native Americans. Public Law 93-638 Contracting and Compacting. https://www.doi.gov/ost/tribal_beneficiaries/contracting. Accessed January 7, 2016.
34. Shore JH, Bloom JD, Manson SM, Whitener RJ. Telemental Health with rural American Indians: issues in civil commitments. Behavioral Sciences and the Law. 2008;26(3):287–300.
35. Yellowlees P, Marks S, Hilty D, et al. Using e-health to enable culturally appropriate mental healthcare in rural areas. Telemedicine Journal and e-Health. 2008;14(5):486–492.
36. Wilshire, T. Telemental health services at a tribally run behavioral health clinic. Psychological Services. 2012;9:318–319.
37. Berwick DM, Nolan TW, Whittington J. The triple aim: care, health, and cost. Health Aff (Milwood). 2008;27(3):759–769.

Telemental Health in Latin America and the Caribbean

TAMMI-MARIE PHILLIP

OVERVIEW OF THE REGION

The Caribbean and Latin America represent a uniquely diverse region whose member countries differ in geographical and population sizes, racial profiles, languages spoken, socioeconomic status, and of course, cultural practices. Within the English-speaking Caribbean alone, countries vary between landlocked masses such as Guyana with an area of 83,000 square miles and a population of predominantly East Indian descent, to St. Kitts and Nevis, 104 square miles in area, and where over 90% of the estimated 55,000 population are of African descent. This great variation in the racial and cultural differences that exist between countries of this region is a direct result of colonization by the big colonial powers—United Kingdom, Spain, France, Portugal and the Netherlands, laying claim to this area. To add to this complexity, many countries changed ownership a number of times, leading to a uniquely distinct culture existing within each country, no matter the size. When you factor in the Latin American region, one can only begin to imagine how diverse of an area this is, and the unique advantages and limitations that this diversity presents.

HISTORY OF MENTAL ILLNESS IN THE CARIBBEAN

To provide a framework on which one can begin to assess avenues to increase access to mental health services in a region that historically has poor mental health service, one needs to first examine the history of mental health and mental illness within this region. Similar to the British model, asylums were established in the late 1800s to keep the mentally ill separate from the rest of society.[1] As psychotherapy improved and more effective treatments were developed, the Caribbean followed the deinstitutionalization model common to the more developed regions of the world.[1] However, due to a number of reasons, this process occurred much slower in the Caribbean region, and this resulted in the highly centralized mental health system, with limited outpatient and community-based mental health resources, that exists today.

Overview of the State of Mental Health in the Caribbean and Latin America

Starting with the Caribbean and moving into Latin America, the following paragraphs will provide an overview of mental health issues and available resources and services.

THE CARIBBEAN

According to a report published by the World Health Organization (WHO) in 2011, "mental and neurological disorders account for almost one-quarter of the total burden of disease in Latin America and the Caribbean." However, within the Caribbean region, the "average percentage of the health budget dedicated to mental health from four-teen countries assessed is 4.33%" with only "four countries receiving more than 5% and seven countries receiving less than 3%."[2] In fact, there has been recent data suggesting that this is an overestimate, and that the actual percentage of health expenditure on mental health is closer to 2%.[2] Interestingly enough, many of the nations spend the majority of their mental health budget on their centralized mental health institutions. This sets up an interesting dilemma because by not adequately appropriating much-needed funds to outpatient facilities, a significant proportion of the population suffering from mental illness is not able to access effective and appropriate care.[2]

The small numbers of mental health professionals, defined as psychia-trists, psychologists, nurses, social workers, and occupational therapists, has historically been, and continues to be, a major road block to the deliv-ery of mental healthcare to those in need. The Caribbean region and Latin America are no exceptions. Per a WHO-AIMS report published in 2011, within the Caribbean region alone, there is a median of 51.7 mental health professionals per 100,000 population.[2] Although this figure may seem large, it is worth noting that there are a number of islands with popula-tions less than 100,000. Within this setting, when looking at the numbers of psychiatrists per 100,000 population, the non-Latin Caribbean has a median of 1.9 psychiatrists.[2] There are also a number of smaller coun-tries with no in-country psychiatrists who rely on solely psychologists and nurses to meet all mental health needs. One of the major setbacks and barriers to increasing the numbers of mental health professionals within this region is the fact that the majority of the countries do not have train-ing programs, and those pursing additional training in psychiatry usually have to seek it outside of the region.[2]

The geographic location of the psychiatrists in these regions is also a consideration, as psychiatrists tend to be concentrated in the urban areas.[2] Of note, this does not pose a major problem to some of the smaller non-Latin Caribbean countries, and this discrepancy may be more of a barrier in the larger countries of Latin America.

Latin America

Similar to the figures reported above, the countries in Latin America allocate a disproportionately low percentage of their total health budget to mental health. Within the eight countries included in the WHO-AIMS report from Latin America in 2013, "the mental health budget as a percentage of the total budget ranged from 0.2% to 7% with a median of 2.05%. In the six countries of Central America, Mexico, and the Latin Caribbean, it ranged from 0.4% to 2.9% with a median of 0.9%."[3] As seen in the Caribbean region, most of the countries within Latin America allocate over 50% of their mental health budget to psychiatric hospitals, leaving very little funding for outpatient facilities.[3]

As discussed in the previous section, inadequate numbers of mental health professionals is also one of the major setbacks to increasing accessibility to mental health services within the Latin American countries. Within Central America, Mexico, and the Latin Caribbean the median number of mental health professionals per 100,000 population is 10.7 (range 6–79) and 26.6 (range 4–173) within South America.[3] The number of psychiatrists per 100,000 population is comparable to that of the non-Latin region with a median of 1.5 (range 0.3–10).[3]

TELEHEALTH IN THE CARIBBEAN AND LATIN AMERICA

To date, although telemental health is not currently employed as a means of increasing access to mental health services, telehealth has taken hold and centers have popped up in some of the islands of the Caribbean. The islands of Saint Lucia, Barbados, The Bahamas, St. Vincent and the Grenadines, Trinidad and Tobago, and Jamaica have recently partnered up with the Hospital for Sick Children in Toronto to improve survival rates for children with hematologic and oncologic diseases through the telehealth modality.[4] While some of the countries had preexisting telemedicine rooms, most of these were located at great distances from the hospital, making them difficult to access. Through this project, telemedicine rooms were either created or upgraded in these countries to "promote and facilitate bi-directional academic exchange both within the Caribbean region and between Caribbean and SickKids" in an effort to "close the gap in childhood survival between low and high resource settings."[5]

Latin America has also extensively explored telehealth as a means of increasing care, and many projects have been researched, developed, and implemented in a number of countries including Brazil, Costa Rica, Chile, and Peru, to name a few. One example of the more active telehealth programs is the Telemedicine University Network (RUTE) developed in 2006 by the Ministry of Science and Technology of Brazil. The RUTE program serves "to expand and consolidate existing telemedicine networks in the country by providing connectivity, informatics and communications teams."[6] By 2011, the RUTE program expanded to 36 telehealth centers and hosted daily videoconferences across a number of medical subspecialties including cardiology, oncology, and child and adolescent health.[6]

The examples of telehealth projects presented above represent a small percentage of those that are currently employed within the Latin American and Caribbean region. Although it does not appear that these telehealth projects have been extended to mental health, these ventures show that this mode of treatment can be a realistic and viable method of increasing access to effective care at a reduced cost.

BENEFITS OF TELEMENTAL HEALTH
IN THE CARIBBEAN AND LATIN AMERICA

One of the major appeals of telemental health is its ability not only to reach persons who would otherwise not seek out mental health due to the associated stigma but also to reach persons who would be unable to access mental healthcare due to physical limitations, whether it be due to the patient's condition or geographical limitations. As discussed in the previous sections, the majority of mental health facilities are located in the major cities. Persons living in rural areas, even in the geographically smaller countries, may find it difficult to make the commute to the cities to receive their mental healthcare. Many may not have the resources to pay for transportation into the major cities, and many of the countries discussed in this chapter have poor public transportation networks that make commuting quite challenging. Coupled with the associated stigma, actively seeking out mental health resources becomes a great challenge that many persons may not wish to undertake, no matter how great the need is. Telemental health provisions could help to overcome these limitations. By having satellite sites in the rural areas, or even systems set up in individual homes, persons may be more proactive in not only seeking out much-needed care but also being advocates for their own mental health.

Although major strides have been made to decrease the stigma associated with mental illness in the Caribbean and Latin America, seeking treatment for mental illness continues to be highly stigmatized within these regions. Given that many of these countries rely heavily on their mental health hospitals as a means to provide treatment to the entire population, persons with less severe mental illness, who would be better served as outpatients, actively refuse mental health treatment to prevent being associated with what many refer to as the country's "crazy house" or "mad house." Even in those countries that do have an outpatient mental health system, given the small population and geographic size of some of the islands within this region, many persons do not seek out treatment in the fear of a peer, colleague, or family member associating them with mental health treatment in some form. Although there exists much work to be done to break down these barriers and reduce the stigma associated with mental health, the provision of telemental health services may help to alleviate this barrier to accessing care. Many more persons may actively seek out mental health treatment if they could do so from discreet locations or even from the comfort of their own homes.

Following along the lines of the stigma associated with mental illness and the small population and geographical sizes of some of the countries explored, one also needs to examine the provider–patient relationship, which as we know, is essential in the treatment of mental health disorders.

It is not uncommon that one of the major barriers to persons receiving mental health treatment is related to either having a personal relationship with the provider or knowing someone who does. Despite mental health records being protected, the few degrees of separation may prevent many persons not only from forming a therapeutic relationship with their provider but also, in many cases, from even seeking treatment. In extreme cases, those patients with significant resources may even resort to receiving their mental health treatment on other islands or countries in an attempt to ensure that their confidentiality be respected. By having treatment providers whom patients do not know personally based in other countries, the therapeutic bond between a patient and their provider, an essential link, may be improved.

Not only would telemental health improve access to general mental health services but also it would allow for access to specialists, which may be nonexistent or very limited in some of the countries within this region. It is not uncommon, especially within the Caribbean region, that patients have to either fly to another country to get specialized medical care, or wait until specialists visit their islands from neighboring countries. As can be imagined, such arrangements are quite costly and are usually not covered by insurance companies. It can also lead to great delays in treating conditions requiring acute interventions. Mental health is no different, and as described above, it is not unheard of for persons with significant resources to fly to different islands to receive specialized mental healthcare. Given that the majority of the populations do not have access to such substantial means, many persons go untreated or are inadequately treated by an already stressed mental health system. One such example is in the field of child and adolescent psychiatry, where the majority of the islands of the Caribbean do not have resident child and adolescent psychiatrists, and children are usually treated by adult psychiatrists or nurses with mental health training. Provision of telemental health would not only allow patients to receive their treatment in their home countries, saving significant amounts of resources, but also allow access to the more specialized and effective treatments that would otherwise not be provided.

LIMITATIONS OF TELEMENTAL HEALTH IN
THE CARIBBEAN AND LATIN AMERICA

Although the provision of telemental health would provide invaluable benefits in the way of cost reduction, improved access to care, and increased access to specialized care, there exist many limitations that would make its implementation difficult at best.

Many of the limitations that exist are the same as those in developed regions such as the United States of America, but given the makeup of the regions explored in this chapter, there are a few unique limitations as well. Cost remains one of the most significant barriers to the implementation of telemental health services within the Caribbean and Latin American regions. Implementing telemental health facilities and infrastructure within the Caribbean and Latin America would most likely require even greater resources than the estimates provided within the United States for a few reasons. One of the major draws of telemental health is increased access to mental health services for those living in rural regions. Not only the cost of the videoconferencing equipment needs to be taken into consideration but also the cost of providing the telephone, Internet service, physical structures, and in some cases even electricity to these locations that are not otherwise connected. Given that spending on mental health is quite low, access to additional funding to implement the necessary infrastructure, although not impossible to obtain, would present a significant challenge, and much of it would have to be outsourced from other regions.

Another major limiting factor in the implementation of telemental health services is the lack of human resources required to make such an endeavor effective. Mental health professionals, in particular psychiatrists, are few and far between. In order to increase access to mental healthcare, more professionals will need to be recruited, which may prove to be particularly challenging, especially in those countries that not do have their own tertiary education institutions and training facilities.

One also needs to consider the training that is needed to efficiently and appropriately provide mental healthcare through telehealth modalities. Not only will adequate training need to be provided for the mental health professionals providing the care, but also for the patients receiving the care. This training would most likely have to be outsourced from developed regions where telemental health is an established means of providing care. The logistics of this could prove to be very difficult to provide on a budget already stretched to the maximum.

Another limitation quite unique to this region is the fact that the Caribbean and Latin America comprise many different countries that, as described above, differ in geographical and population size, racial distribution, and languages spoken. Added to this is the fact that all of the countries, although similar in many respects, also have their own unique cultures. Given that the most efficacious mental health treatment relies on the formation of a therapeutic bond between providers and patients, having providers from different areas within the region may hinder the formation of this therapeutic relationship due to the many differences that exist. Following on this point, considering the "newness" of this mode of mental health treatment provision, one also needs to consider how open patients will be to receiving mental healthcare not only from someone located at times in a different country but also via videoconferencing technology.

One also needs to consider the licensing of the mental health professionals providing the treatment, a problem experienced by other developed countries such as the United States. Providing treatment in a region made up of a number of independent countries poses a significant licensing challenge. How this would work will take much collaboration between the countries and would require the formulation, development, and implementation of discreet guidelines by which telemental health can be effectively practiced.

FUTURE DIRECTIONS

Given that telemental health is one of the major avenues through which mental health treatment can become more accessible, diverse, and cost-effective, a thorough analysis of potential future directions is warranted.

Cost, related not only to the infrastructure but also to the training, remains one of the most significant concerns related to the development of telemental health both in high-income and developing countries. To combat this, more research needs be done to develop cost-effective technologies that can be extended to much of the population. Variations of this have been seen in some of the telehealth projects developed in Latin America, where, for example, cell phones are being used in the treatment of diseases such as HIV.[7] Given the time and resources it would take to develop cheaper technology, another solution would be to develop telemental health facilities at thriving community health centers in the more rural regions. This not only would allow for decreased cost by way of reducing the infrastructure needed but also could lead to improved care coordination, with patients receiving the majority of their medical and psychiatric care in one location.

The patient's comfort and acceptance of this mode of treatment also needs to be taken into consideration when developing a telemental health system. Given that mental health is already highly stigmatized in this region, one could assume that treatment through this modality may impart an additional barrier needed to be overcome by mental health providers. With that being said, this is purely speculation, as to date, not much research, if any, has been conducted looking at the attitudes of patients in this region receiving their psychiatric care through video-conferencing means. Also, given that telehealth has proven to be an effective tool in medical treatment in many of the countries in this region as discussed in previous sections, one can infer that telemental health may also be accepted. Along those lines, focus should be placed on raising public awareness to this form of treatment. The stigma surrounding mental health has decreased over the past few years with the advent of more public mental health awareness campaigns, and one can conclude that similar results may be possible if these campaigns also included telemental health as an avenue to provide treatment.

Lack of human resources, as in many regions, continues to be a barrier to increased access to mental health services. Given that many of the countries within the Caribbean region do not have their own professional schools, the numbers of mental health professionals produced in this region remains low and is inadequate to meet the demands of the population. Forming relationships with institutions, hospitals, and academic centers outside of this region may help to facilitate access to increased numbers of professionals. Exchange programs could be developed where mental health professionals from regions where telemental health is prevalent would not only provide clinical care but also provide the training necessary for the effective delivery of telemental health treatment. Although this would bring up considerations surrounding licensing of mental health practitioners, health policies could be implemented to tackle such issues.

CONCLUSION

This chapter presents an in-depth look at the potential for telemental health within the diverse region of Latin America and the Caribbean. Although this mode of treatment has not been tapped into as of yet, given the fact that telehealth has taken hold, one can infer that telemental health will be one of the major avenues leading to increased access to mental health treatment to those who need it the most.

REFERENCES

1. Hickling FW The history of Caribbean psychiatry. In: Hickling FW, Sorel E, eds. Images of psychiatry: the Caribbean. Kingston, Jamaica: University of the West Indies; 2005.
2. PAHO. WHO-AIMS report on mental health systems in the Caribbean region 2011. http://www.who.int/mental_health/evidence/mh_systems_caribbeans_en.pdf
3. PAHO. WHO-AIMS: report on mental health systems in Latin America and the Caribbean. 2013. http://www.paho.org/hq/index.php?option=com_docman&task=doc_view&gid=21325&Itemid=270
4. Sandals. Sandals Foundation opens first telemedicine room at Victoria Hospital. 2014. http://www.sandalsfoundation.org/news/sandals-foundation-opens-the-first-telemedicine-room-at-victoria-hospital-in-st-lucia.html?article2pdf=1

5. Gillis G, Newsham D, Maeder AJ. Global telehealth 2015: integrating technology and information for better healthcare. Vol 209: Amsterdam, IOS Press; 2015.

6. Oviedo E, Fernández A. e-Health in Latin America and the Caribbean: progress and challenges. United Nations, July 2011. United Nations, Santiago, Chile 2011.

7. Feder JL. Cell-phone medicine brings care to patients in developing nations. Health Affairs. 2010;29(2):259–263.

13

Cross-Cultural Telemental Health

NIKLAS SKOV PAPE, RASMUS CHRISTIAN JØRGENSEN,
AND RUNE WEISE KOFOED

Cross-cultural research in relation to telemental health is still in its infancy and a rather unexplored field. Further research on this topic is seen by some researchers as increasingly significant as the need to treat patients suffering from mental illness and especially unipolar depression is expected to grow in the coming decades.[1,2] Using modern information and communications technology (ICT) and telepsychiatric instruments in treatment across cultures could be seen as a promising solution for helping patients in low- and middle-income countries.[3,4] This approach, however, also comes with an additional need for a thorough understanding of intercultural considerations, which is what we address in this chapter. First we discuss the cross-cultural aspect of the patient–doctor relationship and subsequently address the aspects and issues of a sociotechnological view of development and implementation of telepsychiatry across cultures. Lastly we summarize with some concluding considerations.

PSYCHOPATHOLOGICAL CONCEPTS AND
THE IMPORTANCE OF A CROSS-CULTURAL
UNDERSTANDING OF MENTAL HEALTH

The cultural setting is in some ways a defining aspect of humans as individuals. It can affect whether the best practice for a person with a mental illness would be to seek help from a psychiatrist, the local priest, a wise elderly, or perhaps a witchdoctor. It also defines how we are perceived among friends, families, and other people in general, for example, when we are experiencing sickness. To understand why we need to know about cultural aspects when working with telemental health across cultures, let us start with a basic understanding of the notion of health and how some studies actually find that the concept of health differs across cultures.

The term "disease" refers to a health problem that consists of a physiological malfunction resulting in an actual or potential reduction in physical capacity and/or reduced life expectancy. The term "illness" refers to the human experience and perception of a physical malfunction. Illness is the subjectively interpreted undesirable state of ill-health, based on general explanations of a given sickness.[5] The term "sickness" refers to "the society's way of making sense of and dealing with the individual perception of malfunctioning (illness); and the underlying pathology (disease).[5(p. 408)] None of these states demands the presence of the others, as it is possible for an individual to subjectively experience illness without the presence of an actual disease and it is also possible that an individual is the victim of a given disease, without experiencing illness.[6]

> Psychosocial factors have been increasingly recognized as key factors in the success of health and social actions. If actions are to be effective in the prevention of disease and in the promotion of health and wellbeing, they must be based on an understanding of culture, tradition, beliefs and patterns of family interaction.[7(p 4)]

From a cross-cultural perspective, it is safe to say that an understanding of distinctions and cultural differences in perceived illness and social acceptance of mental disorders is crucial when researching differences in health and help-seeking behaviors in developing countries. This is not only because what is regarded as a disease by Western biomedicine may carry rather different meanings in non-Western communities[8] but also because local health concepts and phrases used to describe syndromes appear different in some societies.[9] As the diagnostic process is highly dependent on the individual's ability to express his or her thoughts and feelings, it is of paramount importance that the mental health workers in question have a sufficient understanding of the given patient's culture and social setting.

These points, the aforementioned findings, and recent research collectively tell us that for a cross-cultural psychiatric treatment, consultation, or diagnosis to be successful, it is crucial that the mental health workers in question have at least some understanding of the culture and norms of the patient's society, as well as an understanding of the given society's view on mental illness.[5(pp405-429)] Yet, it is important to note that the cultural novice or psychiatrist who has little knowledge of his patient's culture and little time to learn much more about it, can still do culturally sensitive and appropriate work.

According to an evaluation of the use of the Cultural Consultation Service in Canada, conducted by Kirmayer, Groleau, and Rousseau,[10] the use of what they call cultural consultants, culture brokers, and interpreters often helped clinicians identify important social and cultural issues that could potentially influence treatment and constitute important clinical problems. Furthermore, it was found that referring clinicians generally found the service helpful for understanding the complex cases and that the cultural consultations can improve treatment engagement and adherence. It is carefully estimated that the use of cultural consultation can indeed have a dramatic impact on individual cases.[10]

In regard to the potential use of telepsychiatric measures in developing countries, the understanding of local concepts of mental illness and specific syndromes is needed. Bass, Bolton, and Murray pointed out that this understanding is essential not only to develop a locally appropriate study instrument that can be used for measurement of prevalence and incidence of illness and evaluation of the effectiveness of innovative intervention strategies (e.g., telemental health or telepsychiatry) but also later in the actual telepsychiatric process.[9]

Despite differences in the distinctions of health phenomena across cultures, "culture-bound syndromes," a term for local patterns of behavior that do not fit into the Western psychiatric classification, has been called a redundant term, as all reactions are to some extent culturally determined.[8] Nevertheless, this classification helps us understand health phenomena that are restricted to a limited number of cultures on the basis of psychosocial features. In regard to our focus on cross-cultural telepsychiatric treatment, this is important, as the Western psychiatrist otherwise would risk falling under what the American psychiatrist and researcher Arthur Kleinman called the *category fallacy*, which implies the limitations of these studies based on prevalence rates.[11] By imputing the illness categories of his or her own culture to the patient's culture, the psychiatrist, in this case sitting in another part of the world, could risk making erroneous assumptions and thereby misdiagnosing the patient—which could then precariously lead to, for instance, inadequate therapy or prescribing the wrong medication.

THE EXAMPLE OF DEPRESSION, DIAGNOSTIC DIFFERENCES AND CULTURAL VARIATIONS

It is worth mentioning that some researchers claim that there is still not sufficient evidence to support actual differences in major psychiatric disorders across cultures and societies[12] and that descriptions of a mental illness developed in one set of cultures are in fact equally applicable to other foreign cultures.[13] Nevertheless, alongside the establishment of the subdisciplinary study of cultural differences in psychopathology, commonly known as comparative psychiatry, the field of cross-cultural psychotherapy has become aware of the potential consequences of an uncritical application of standard diagnostic criteria across cultures,[5(pp 422-423),13] implying that if the nature of emotions, thoughts, and behaviors are culturally variable, diagnostics made on standard Western psychotherapeutic criteria could potentially lead to misleading or erroneous results[14]—even though the depressive syndrome, for instance, has later been claimed to be remarkably similar throughout a wide range of languages, cultures, and economic wealth.[13]

Some researchers within the field of cross-cultural understanding of depression also claim that differential depression diagnosis across cultures is likely not to exist,[15] suggesting that depression is a seemingly consistent phenomenon throughout the world. Similarly, later studies showed that cross-cultural diagnostic differences disappeared when patients were diagnosed on the basis of the World Health Organization's (WHO's) standardized diagnostic system (ICD-8).[15(p758)] However, earlier studies concluded that no universal conception of depression exists, though variants of depressive disorders similar to those in Western cultures sometimes have been found among cultures without a conceptual equivalent.[15] As an example of a variation, several studies conducted over a course of more than 20 years, have shown that the sense of guilt has emerged as a source of cultural variation among the symptoms of depression.[15(p762)] Studies have shown that patients in low-income countries with limited knowledge of the Western understanding of mental disorders experience somatizations in relation to depressive disorders.[13] Lastly, Cox[16] and Cheng[17] have both pointed out the importance of ensuring the semantic or psycholinguistic equivalents of the psychiatric symptoms across cultures, before psychopathological diagnostic instruments can be operationalized, and we believe that this is equally important to take into account when implementing telepsychiatric measures across cultures. Telepsychiatric measures therefore constitute a culturally sensitive practice, and it is necessary and important to adapt these measures to the local cultures instead of just exporting Western models.

IMPORTANT CULTURAL ISSUES
IN TELEMENTAL HEALTH

As discussed, there are indeed important cultural issues and implications to consider when implementing telemental health in a cross-cultural setting. Culturally appropriate care has been pointed out as an essential, if not crucial, component of telemental health in regard to process and outcome.[18] Studies show that cultural understanding is becoming an increasingly larger part of the patient–doctor relationship within the use of telepsychiatry. However, to this day there still does not exist a systematic framework clearly addressing cultural issues of telepsychiatry.[9,18]

Using telemental health across borders and cultures entails obvious barriers, such as language, trust, technological knowledge and experience, and potential unfamiliarity with the patient's cultural setting. These examples are all issues that have been accentuated as important subjects for further research in the field of telemental health.[18] As previously stated, differences in local health concepts demand the involved psychiatrist's attention, as the given setting creates the psychosocial context through which the patient will express feelings and thoughts.[5,9,14] Again, it is clear that cultural insight and understanding constitute an essential characteristic to a successful treatment through telemental health services.

A group of researchers involved in telepsychiatric studies and tests with both North American Indian communities and Alaskan native elders published a study dealing with the cultural issues of telepsychiatry within these relatively secluded, rural communities. The research group presents a list of issues that future providers of telepsychiatry are encouraged to take into account. These issues include inquiring about the patient's level of comfort with technology, becoming familiar with and adapting to local communication styles, and assessing the patient's understanding and feelings toward confidentiality and the implications of telepsychiatry for their confidentiality.[18] These examples are a just few of the issues we believe are important to take into account when potentially implementing a telepsychiatric solution across cultures and borders. By including these points, we encourage researchers and practitioners to conduct further studies and projects within this particular field and context, because we have found that the field of telemental health and the importance of a cross-cultural aspect, as an interrelated entity, generally lacks research. This is supported by Shore et al.,[18] who describe difficulty in finding existing articles on the subject of cultural appropriateness or cultural competency in telemental health specifically.

APPROACHING CULTURAL BARRIERS IN DEVELOPMENT
AND IMPLEMENTATION OF TELEMENTAL HEALTH

Earlier we presented and discussed cultural differences in psychopathology as one crucial fragment of the many cross-cultural challenges and barriers concerning implementation of telemental health in low- and middle-income countries. Here we identify the need for alternative approaches to fathom these nontechnical issues. These cross-cultural barriers are not in themselves a technical matter. Instead they are social, related to questions about society and the specific contextual setting. Within the field of diffusion and adoption—the academic and professional field concerning how new technology spreads and anchors within the user groups—a sociotechnical approach is blooming to embrace the colors, shades, and dimensions of the social aspects of adoption, diffusion, and implementation of ICTs.

In regard to telemental health, we argue there definitely is both a technological and a social dimension, and the two cannot be clearly separated. The technical dimension is the hard-system development—ER-diagramming, data modeling, programming, and so forth—in other words, the hard design of the system. But when considering design, use, implementation, adoption, and diffusion, we argue for the necessity to mainly focus on the social aspects, to address the cross-cultural challenges—for example, the contrasting understanding of psychopathology across cultures. With a sociotechnical approach, projects and research would be provided with the necessary tools and techniques—and importantly the focus—to embrace the social dimensions and thereby address the potential cultural barriers of the application and use of telemental health in developing countries.

As earlier stated, there is to date no sufficient framework for development or implementation of telemental health technology. We suggest that future development of a framework needs to focus and carefully bring attention to a sociotechnical understanding for greater sufficiency, applicability, and utility. A "one-size-fits-all" universal model, that is capable of containing and relating all social and technical aspects (and then even across cultures) might be an impossible and utopian goal. But if the framework were developed as a framework and not as a guide, tool, or technique (as often is the case with so-called frameworks) and from the beginning focused on constant dynamic development and ongoing iterations closely connected to actual practice and experience, it might be more likely that the framework would be able to fathom the wide range of social and technical dimensions of implementation of telemental health across cultures. To put it another way, the framework should be adapted and developed in relation to the given context, instead of trying to make the context fit the framework.

CONCLUSION

The objective of this chapter was to expound and discuss previous experiences with telemental health as well as research regarding the importance of cross-cultural understanding of mental health, but more importantly, the potential psychological barriers within a cross-cultural telepsychiatric treatment in low- and middle-income countries.

With concern, we find that the cross-cultural aspect between patients and therapists is almost absent in recent research on telemental health, as the majority of studies regarding telemental health to this day have been conducted solely in Western countries. This has also been pointed out by Chipps et al.[19] This is an obvious worry because patients' health beliefs, attitudes, and behaviors are rooted in their specific cultural setting, and failing to consider this can have negative consequences for patients. It is exceedingly important that the involved mental health workers at some degree have an appropriate understanding of both the cultural background and psychosocial environment of the patients they serve.

The need for further research in the area of telemedicine and telemental health is critical as it will increase the credibility of the field by demonstrating cost effectiveness and impact on clear clinical outcomes.[3,20,21]

It is argued that a focus on a sociotechnical approach in developing a dynamic, iterative, and flexible framework for telemental health could increase its sufficiency, applicability, and utility by striving to include social, human, cultural, and technological aspects, and ultimately could provide practitioners (both technical and healthcare) with a necessary and much needed system for development and implementation of telemental health.

It is important to disrupt what seems to be a dichotomy among researchers between telemental health and cross-cultural psychology in order to ensure better and safer consultations across cultures when using telemental health solutions.

REFERENCES

1. Mathers C, Fat D, Boerma J. The global burden of disease. Geneva, Switzerland: World Health Organization; 2008.
2. Murray C, Lopez A. Alternative projections of mortality and disability by cause 1990–2020: Global burden of disease study. Lancet. 1997;349(9064):1498–1504. doi:10.1016/s0140-6736(96)07492-2.
3. Wootton R, Bonnardot L. In what circumstances is telemedicine appropriate in the developing world? JRSM Short Reports. 2010;1(5):37–37. doi:10.1258/shorts.2010.010045.
4. Chipps J, Brysiewicz P, Mars M. Effectiveness and feasibility of telepsychiatry in resource constrained environments? A systematic review of the evidence. African Journal of Psychiatry. 2012;15(4). doi:10.4314/ajpsy.v15i4.30.
5. Berry J. Cross-cultural psychology. Cambridge: Cambridge University Press; 2011.
6. Kleinman A, Eisenberg L, Good B. Culture, illness, and care: clinical lessons from anthropologic and cross-cultural research. FOC. 2006;4(1):140–149. doi:10.1176/foc.4.1.140.
7. The WHO Medium-Term Mental Health Programme 1975–1982. Interim Report. Geneva: World Health Organisation: WHO; 1982.
8. Littlewood R. From categories to contexts: a decade of "the new cross-cultural psychiatry." British Journal of Psychiatry. 1990;156(3):308–327. doi:10.1192/bjp.156.3.308.
9. Bass J, Bolton P, Murray L. Do not forget culture when studying mental health. Lancet. 2007;370(9591):918–919. doi:10.1016/s0140-6736(07)61426-3.
10. Kirmayer L, Groleau D, Rousseau C. Development and evaluation of the cultural consultation service. Cultural Consultation. 2013;21–45. doi:10.1007/978-1-4614-7615-3_2.
11. Kleinman A. Depression, somatization and the "new cross-cultural psychiatry." Social Science and Medicine (1967). 1977;11(1):3–9. doi:10.1016/0037-7856(77)90138-x.
12. Cheng A. Case definition and culture: are people all the same? British Journal of Psychiatry. 2001;179(1):1–3. doi:10.1192/bjp.179.1.1.
13. Simon G, Goldberg D, Von Korff M, Üstün T. Understanding cross-national differences in depression prevalence. Psychological Medicine. 2002;32(04). doi:10.1017/s0033291702005457.

14. Kleinman A. Rethinking psychiatry: from cultural category to personal experience. New York: Bulletin of Science, Technology and Society; 1988;8(4):454–454. doi:10.1177/0270467688008004133.

15. Draguns J, Tanaka-Matsumi J. Assessment of psychopathology across and within cultures: issues and findings. Behaviour Research and Therapy. 2003;41(7):755–776. doi:10.1016/s0005-7967(02)00190-0.

16. Cox J. Aspects of transcultural psychiatry. British Journal of Psychiatry. 1977;130(3):211–221. doi:10.1192/bjp.130.3.211.

17. Cheng T. Symptomatology of minor psychiatric morbidity: a crosscultural comparison. Psychological Medicine. 1989;19(03):697. doi:10.1017/s0033291700024296.

18. Shore J, Savin D, Novins D, Manson S. Cultural aspects of telepsychiatry. J Telemed Telecare. 2006;12(3):116–121. doi:10.1258/135763306776738602.

19. Chipps J, Brysiewicz P, Mars M. Effectiveness and feasibility of telepsychiatry in resource constrained environments? A systematic review of the evidence. Afr J Psych. 2012;15(4). doi:10.4314/ajpsy.v15i4.30.

20. Ryu S. Telemedicine: opportunities and developments in member states: report on the second global survey on ehealth 2009 (Global Observatory for eHealth Series, Volume 2). Healthc Inform Res. 2012;18(2):153. doi:10.4258/hir.2012.18.2.153.

21. Monnier J, Knapp R, Frueh B. Recent advances in telepsychiatry: an updated review. PS. 2003;54(12):1604–1609. doi:10.1176/appi.ps.54.12.1604.

14

Telemental Health in Postdisaster Settings

EUGENE F. AUGUSTERFER, RICHARD F. MOLLICA,
AND JAMES LAVELLE

Telemental health (TMH) and telemedicine are important components in meeting critical health and mental health needs of the global population, including those who have suffered from natural disasters or from man-made or technological disasters. The need for mental health services to address the trauma caused by disasters is well documented. Over 1 billion persons (1 in 6) worldwide have been affected by natural disasters and/or armed conflict.[1] Natural disasters and armed conflict have marked human existence throughout history and have always caused peaks in mortality and morbidity. But in recent times, the scale and scope of these events have increased markedly. Since 1990, natural disasters have affected about 217 million people every year.[2]

Mental health is an issue of global importance; accounting for 13% of the global disease burden.[3] Telemental health and telemedicine promise to bring much-needed specialty expertise to those in postdisaster and difficult-to-reach settings.

This chapter discusses the impact of disasters—natural, man-made, and technological—on the health and mental health of survivors and the role of TMH in meeting the ongoing needs of disaster survivors.

Countries or settings that have suffered natural disasters such as floods, earthquakes, hurricanes, or droughts often have damaged or destroyed vital systems, such as security, economic, health, and welfare systems. While there are many examples, a good example of the impact of a natural disaster is the 2010 Haiti earthquake, which caused loss of life, massive destruction, and displacement of over a million people. Survivors of natural disasters face numerous obstacles to recovery, including health and mental health problems. Later in this chapter, we examine these issues in depth.

Postconflict settings are similar to post-natural-disaster settings in that vital systems such as security, economic, health, and welfare institutions have often been damaged or destroyed, increasing instability in the society. However, an important distinction is that in postconflict settings there is the knowledge that someone inflicted the trauma by choice. This has lasting impact on the society and impacts recovery efforts.

IMPACT OF DISASTERS

Natural disasters are on the rise worldwide as documented by the Centre for Research on the Epidemiology of Disasters,[4] as a consequence, humanitarian, health, and mental health needs for postdisaster relief are on the rise as well. By the end of 2015, the Office of the United Nations High Commissioner for Refugees counted 65.3 million forcibly displaced people worldwide, with the majority of the displaced people coming from low- and middle-income countries (LMICs).[5]

The need for health and mental health services to address the problems caused by disasters is well documented. Depression is leading cause of disability worldwide, and is a major contributor to the overall global burden of disease.[6]

"Disasters, terrorism and traumatic events, whatever their source or scale, bring with them the potential to cause distress. Every person who is directly or indirectly involved in such an event may be affected and many may need psychosocial support."[7] During and following a disaster, it is difficult for individuals and families, who are suddenly thrown into unfamiliar situations as much of what they have known—homes, work, schools, and so forth—is damaged and/or destroyed. Loss of life of a loved one, friend, or neighbor and/or injury to self, a friend, or neighbor increases the sense of "unreality" in the acute postdisaster phase. In addition to the medical care that might be needed for physical injuries, it is not surprising that great numbers of survivors develop trauma-related mental health problems. As discussed in this chapter, TMH and telemedicine have the capacity to enable health professionals from around the world to assist local health and mental health personnel in postdisaster settings, but first we examine the impact of disasters on the mental health of survivors.

MENTAL HEALTH CONSEQUENCES OF DISASTERS

Disasters, both natural and man-made, affect millions of people around the world every year.[8] Although temporary symptoms tend to be common in the acute phase of disaster recovery, psychological sequelae can persist for up to 3 to 5 years after a natural disaster.[9] In recent years, there have been a number of examples of large-scale disasters with multiple etiologies, both natural and man-made. A common thread in all of these disaster events is their significant impact on the health and mental health of survivors. As such, a percentage of the postdisaster population will develop mental health problems, such as, post-traumatic stress disorder (PTSD).

In a systematic review of PTSD following disasters, Neria, Nandi, and Galea examined 284 peer-reviewed published studies of PTSD following disasters, natural, man-made, and technological, and concluded that "PTSD among persons exposed to disasters is substantial" and that the most consistently documented determinants of the risk of PTSD across the studies examined is the magnitude of exposure to the event.[10]

In a study of the Wenchuan earthquake (China), Hong and Efferth found that adolescent and adult survivors had high prevalence rates of PTSD.[11] In a study of the mental health impact of the Great East Japan Earthquake (GEJE), tsunami, and nuclear disaster of 2011, which killed over 15,000 persons and displaced over 300,000 persons from their homes, Tsujiuchi et al. report the rates of PTSD in displaced persons to be in excess of 35%.[12] Sezqin and Punamaki examined social relations of 1,253 women exposed to earthquake trauma in Eastern Anatolia, Turkey, and found that "severe earthquake trauma was associated with deteriorated social relations, especially neighborhood and marital relations. Deteriorated marital and child relations were associated with increased levels of psychiatric distress" including PTSD.[13] In another study of a natural disaster, Tracy, Norris, and Gales examined the survivors of Hurricane Ike, which struck the gulf coast of Texas (United States) in 2008 to assess "the differences in the determinants of PTSD and depression after this event, including the particular hurricane experiences including postevent nontraumatic stressors that were associated with these pathologies. They found that specific hurricane-related stressors such as loss or damage of sentimental possessions were associated with both PTSD and depression. They concluded that PTSD is indeed a disorder of "event exposure," whereas risk of depression is more clearly driven by personal vulnerability and exposure to stressors. The role of nontraumatic stressors in shaping risk of both pathologies suggests that alleviating stressors after disasters has clear potential to mitigate the psychological impact of these events."[14]

In a study of a man-made disaster, Perlman et al. examined the survivors of the New York City terrorist attacks of September 11, 2001 (9/11), in which 2,800 people were killed and thousands more had subsequent health problems. In their review of health effects in the short and medium terms, strong evidence is provided for associations between experiencing or witnessing events related to 9/11 and PTSD and respiratory illness, with a correlation between prolonged, intense exposure and increased overall illness and disability. Risk factors for PTSD included proximity to the site on 9/11, living or working in lower Manhattan, rescue or recovery work at the World Trade Center site, event-related loss of spouse, and low social support.[15] In a study of the armed conflict in Syria, Alpak et al. studied 352 Syrian refugees living in a refugee settlement camp in Turkey and found a frequency rate of 33.5% for PTSD. However, when they examined female refugees who had a previous psychiatric disorder, a family history of a psychiatric disorder, and experienced two or more traumas, the probability of developing PTSD jumped to 71%.[16] In a study of traumatic head injury (THI), Mollica et al. studied the mental health sequelae of Cambodian ex-political detainees who survived torture, and found that those who had suffered THI were much more likely to suffer depression and PTSD.[17] In a study of a Sri Lankan population, a country that has suffered long-term (25+ years) internal armed conflict and a significant natural disaster, the 2004 tsunami, Wickrama, et al found significant mental health impact related to disaster exposure.[18] In a study in an ongoing armed conflict setting, Jefee-Bahloul, Moustafa, Shebl, and Barkil-Oteo surveyed 354 Syrian refugees and reported that 41.8% had scores on HADStress that correlated to PTSD.[19]

In a review of technological disasters, Tsujiuchi et al., as stated previously, examined the mental health impact of the GEJE, a natural and technological disaster (nuclear disaster), and found rates of PTSD in excess of 35%.[12] In another technological disaster, Contis and Foley studied depression, suicidal ideation, and thyroid tumors among Ukrainian adolescents exposed as children to the Chernobyl disaster: 115,191 adolescents were screened for depression, suicide ideation, and psychological problems using the Children's Depression Inventory. Depression was diagnosed in 15,399 adolescents (13.2%), suicide ideation in 813 (5.3%), and attempted suicide in 354 (2.3%). Underlying components of the participants' depression were negative mood, interpersonal difficulties, and negative self-esteem.[20]

Based on a review of the literature, it seems clear that disasters, natural, man-made, and technological, leave in their path death, destruction, physical injury, and emotional suffering. Therefore, treating both the physical and emotional impact of disasters is imperative for the long-term well-being of survivors! Reinforcing the need for addressing the mental health impact of disasters, Boscarino found that a major factor in the mental health recovery of disaster survivors is the availability of mental health and psychosocial resources.[21]

THE NEED FOR SUSTAINABLE CARE

Another important issue to be examined is what is referred to as sustainable care. Olsen defined sustainable healthcare as "a health service operated by an organizational system with the long-term ability to mobilize and allocate sufficient resources for activities that meet individual or public health needs."[22] In the context of disaster response, sustainable care can be defined, in part, by responders staying to provide needed care during the emergency phase and the early stages of recovery. The work of international actors is critical to postdisaster trauma treatment; however, it is also the nature of emergency disaster response that it tends to be geared toward the immediate response dealing with the most acute problems. Experiences, as well as careful observation, reflect the reality that mental health problems tend to surface after the acute phase of disaster recovery, therefore creating a gap between the departure of most disaster response teams and the appearance of mental health problems. Olteanu et al. examined the persistence of mental health needs of children following Hurricane Katrina in New Orleans (United States) and found that "mental health service needs continued unabated throughout the disaster recovery period (two to nearly four years post-event). And, 29% of pediatric primary care patients presented with mental health or developmental/learning problems, including the need for intensive case management."[23]

Given that health and mental health–related problems tend to remain long after the acute phase of disaster recovery, it stands to reason that the mental health response needs to remain after the acute phase. However, the reality is emergency responders are often being asked to move to the next disaster, therefore, availability of mental health care is severely impacted. Given this reality, how does one address the postdisaster ongoing health and mental health problems?

THE ROLE OF TELEMENTAL HEALTH
IN SUSTAINABLE CARE

We now examine the role of telemental health in addressing the important need for sustainable mental healthcare.

As we have seen, it is the nature of disaster emergency response teams to focus efforts on the immediate needs of saving lives, treating the acutely injured following a disaster. However, it is also the nature of these dedicated professionals that they are frequently deployed to the next disaster site following the acute recovery phase. However, as we have documented, mental health problems often surface and remain after the acute phase of postdisaster recovery, creating a gap in services and exposing the need for ongoing and sustainable care.

Telemental health can help fill these gaps with much-needed sustainable mental health services. However, published reports on the use of telemedicine in postdisaster settings are relatively infrequent.[24] One of the first documented uses of telemedicine in disaster response was the 1988 earthquake in Soviet Armenia. Nicogossian and Doarn looked at lessons learned following the earthquake and found that "psychological, physical, and social sequelae persist years after the events." The authors go on to report that telemedicine was useful in response to the needs of survivors and that telemental health would be helpful in targeting the psychological sequelae noted in the report.[25]

Simmons et al. examined the use of telehealth in postdisaster response and found that "telehealth would play primarily a support role in this acute phase and would continue to fill gaps in specialty care services such as mental health. Further, recent advances in high-speed networks can be harnessed for improved triage, teleconsultation, and postevent psychiatric/psychological consultation or long-term patient follow-up.[26]

Yellowlees et al. looked at the use of TMH in emergencies and found that "telepsychiatry (telemental health) can be used in two kinds of psychiatric emergencies: one-time clinical events and public health situations associated with mass disasters," and that telemental health can "improve access to psychiatric care in the event of a natural or man-made disaster."[27]

In a study of survivors of a major bushfire disaster in Australia, Reifels, Bassilios, and Pirkis examined the use of telemental health and found that despite the lack of quantitative data, all three telemental health services that were used (Kids Helpline, MensLine Australia, and Lifeline Australia) "experienced significant increases in overall service uptake levels in the wake of the bushfires."[28]

As we have seen in the literature review, TMH brings the capacity to supplement on-the-ground mental healthcare efforts. The model of collaboration between distant providers and the on-site providers for clinical training, case consultation, supervision, or second opinions has been used successfully and, in the opinion of the authors, can be used in postdisaster settings to augment the need for specialty care.

CASE EXAMPLE: HAITI

On January 12, 2010, a 7.0-magnitude earthquake shook Haiti, with the epicenter only 10 miles from Port-au-Prince, the bustling capital city of the Caribbean country. One of the most destructive natural disasters in history, the quake reduced buildings to rubble, instantly taking lives and destroying homes. The United States Geological Survery (USGS) estimates that 316,000 people died, 300,000 were injured, and over 1.3 million were displaced from their homes.[29] The impact of this devastating event, which caused the aforementioned loss of life, severe damage of property, and displacement of the population also destroyed clinics and hospitals, which were therefore unable to function as medical care centers. However, health and mental healthcare personnel from all over the world joined forces to treat the wounded.

Medical and Mental Health Impact

To better understand the medical and mental health impact of the 2010 earthquake, it is important to understand the overall picture of Haiti. The

World Bank lists Haiti as a low-income country, the poorest country in the Americas, and one of the poorest in the world, with 77% of the population living in poverty.[30]

Prior to the 2010 earthquake, almost half of the population of Haiti had no access to healthcare services because there was no healthcare facility near them.[31] The World Health Organization Mental Health Atlas 2011 reported the majority of physicians in Haiti are PCPs with the majority of mental healthcare being provided by these primary care doctors and nurses. However, the majority of these doctors and nurses have not received official in-service training in mental health within the last 5 years.[32]

As stated earlier, as a result of the earthquake, over 316,000 persons died, over 300,000 were injured, and 1.3 million persons were displaced from their homes, rendering the population in tremendous need and the Haitian healthcare system overwhelmed.

However, when the earthquake struck, there was a rapid international response. Bailey, Bailey, and Akpudo reported on their experience just 2 weeks after the earthquake that the "need for food, shelter, health care, and psychological support among these displaced and devastated people was brutally obvious."[33] McShane wrote about her experience as a psychiatric resident serving in a field hospital and reported that in addition to the loss of life and the destruction of property, Haiti lacked a coordinated mental healthcare system and that "hundreds of patients presented to triage and emergency rooms daily with symptoms related to psychiatric disorders, such as heart palpitations, sweats, headaches, and memory problems."[34] In another study, Cenat and Derivois examined the prevalence and determinants of PTSD and depression symptoms in adult survivors of the earthquake and found of the 1,355 adults (660 women), the prevalence rates of PTSD and depressive symptoms were 36.75% and 25.98% respectively.[35] In a study of the prevalence of PTSD and depression in children 1 year after the 2010 earthquake, Blanc, et al stated that while more than 500 studies were conducted in Haiti following the earthquake, very few assessed the mental health impact on the population. In their study, they found that using the Child Behavior Check-List, more than 50% of the children tested had severe PTSD symptoms. Blanc et al. went on to say that serious attention should be paid to the mental health aspects in the reconstruction program for Haiti.[36]

The authors visited Haiti in April of 2014, more than 4 years after the earthquake, and found that health and mental health services were still lacking. Given the dire situation in Haiti remains, it is important that health and mental health programs be developed to meet the continuing needs with sustainable health and mental healthcare.

The Role of Telemedicine and Telemental Health
in Postdisaster Haiti

Before reviewing the reports on the use of TMH in response to the 2010 Haitian earthquake, it is important to state that due to the earthquake epicenter being close to the capital, Port-au-Prince, much of the infrastructure, including telecommunications, was destroyed or badly damaged. Therefore, TMH and telemedicine were severely hampered due to the lack of telecommunications. However, there were some innovative TMH efforts, which are reviewed in this section.

Louden reported in *Medscape Medical News* that "just days after the devastating earthquake struck Haiti on January 12, medical volunteers from the University of Miami in Florida arrived and set up a tent hospital in Port-au-Prince. Antonio C. Marttos, Jr., of the University of Miami School of Medicine, reported "everything was destroyed over there, and in the first days there was no Internet in Port-au-Prince, but we were able to connect to our trauma center in Miami with the use of satellite for triage and video consultations." Marttos went on, "what's most exciting is that we are building an entire health system in Haiti, including telemedicine."[37] In a study of the use of mobile health (mHealth), Walters reported that in a postdisaster environment, the use of mHealth significantly improved the delivery of care. The results of the study "show that physicians in many different specialties employed telemedicine consultations in a wide range of patients and illnesses. Telemedicine consultations significantly affected the diagnosis in 30%, the treatment in 32%, and the overall patient status in 70% of cases."[38] In another study, Tenq et al. studied the use of mHealth in Haiti's cholera epidemic and found that the use of GPS assisted with management of the data of 50,000 participants in two isolated communities. In doing so, they were able to document the vaccination of 45,417 people receiving at least one dose and 90.8% received a second dose. As such, mHealth technology allowed for the creation of an electronic registry with specific population census data and specific location, thus saving time and energy in the future.[39] While the Tenq study did not use mHealth for mental health, it is worth noting that mHealth is being used as a component of telemental health in other settings.

Finally, in a unique and innovative use of telemedicine, a fisherman from St. Petersburg, Florida, used his ham radio to establish a connection with *USS Comfort*, a US Navy hospital ship, and doctors in Haiti, thus supporting medical care in Haiti, to include the transfer of an imperiled infant to *USS Comfort* for urgent medical care.

SUMMARY AND CONCLUSION

As we have reviewed, disasters, natural, man-made, or technological, cause significant loss of life, injuries and suffering, destruction of property, and displacement of people. The need for medical and mental healthcare is critical. The medical needs of survivors is often addressed promptly, whereas, mental health needs are often not as visible and therefore often overlooked and not addressed. The issue is complicated by the fact that globally LMICs are disproportionately impacted by disasters and the majority of medical providers in these countries are PCPs. While these PCPs do a tremendous job saving lives and addressing acute injuries and illnesses, they often are not trained to recognize and treat mental health related problems. Therefore, it is important to recognize this gap and equally important to develop a system to support PCPs with mental health trauma-related education, training, supervision, and importantly, ongoing peer support. Telemental health should

be an important component of such a comprehensive system by helping bring much-needed specialty expertise in mental health to those
working in postdisaster settings. Studies support the feasibility, acceptability, and effectiveness of TMH; therefore, it should be an important
component in supporting those on the front lines of disaster response.
While telemedicine and TMH have been deployed in postdisaster settings, they remain underused. Further, published articles on the use
of telemedicine and TMH in these settings are lacking. Making this
point, Latifi and Tilley reviewed the literature and found that 17,565
disasters were reported between January 1980 and September 2013 and
878 articles, books, and so forth, reported on the disasters. However,
only 19 articles provided examples of the effective use of telemedicine
in disaster response.[41]

Lastly, while there are a number of challenges that must be overcome
in the implementation of a comprehensive TMH postdisaster response
program, such as educating providers to work in varied cultures, working through translators, time zone differences, and more, the authors
would like to emphasize the importance and great satisfaction of disaster
response work and the important role of TMH in ensuring the delivery of
evidence-based best practices to those in critical need.

REFERENCES

1. Mollica R. Lecture: Global Mental Health: Trauma and Recovery. Orvieto,
    Italy, 2007.
2. Leaning L, Guha-Sapir D. Natural disasters, armed conflict, and public health. New
    England Journal of Medicine. 2013;369:1836–1842.
3. Vigo D, Thornicroft G, Atun R. Estimating the true global burden of mental illness.
    The Lancet, Psychiatry. 2016;3(2):171–178.
4. Disaster Trends. The International Disaster Database, Centre for Research on the
    Epidemiology of Disasters April 2016.
5. United Nations High Commissioner on Refugees. Global Trends in Forced
    Displacement in 2015, June 2016.
6. World Health Organization. Depression Fact sheet, April 2016.
7. Psychosocial Care for People Affected by Disasters and Major Incidents. A Model
    for Disigning, Delivering and Managing Psychosocial Services for People Involved

in Major Incidents, Conflict, Disasters and Terrorism. NATO Joint Medical Committee, September 2008.

8. Rossi PH, Wright JD, Weber-Burdin E, Pereira J. Victimization by natural hazards in the United States, 1970–1980: survey estimates. International Journal of Mass Emergencies and Disasters. 1983;1:467–482.

9. Lima BR, Pai S, Toledo V, et al. Emotional distress in disaster victims: a follow-up study. Journal of Nervous and Mental Disease. 1993;181:388–393.

10. Neria Y, Nandi A, Galea S. Post-traumatic stress disorder following disasters: a systematic review. Psychological Medicine. 2008;38:467–480.

11. Hong C, Efferth T. Systematic review on Post-Traumatic Stress Disorder Among Survivors of the Wenchuan Earthquake, Trauma, Vilence & Abuse. 2016 Dec;17(5):552–561.

12. Tsujiuchi T, Yamaguchi M, Masuda K, et al. High Prevalence of Post-Traumatic Stress Symptons in Relation to Social Factors in Affected Population One Year after the Fukushima Nuclear Disaster. Plos One. 2016 Mar 22;11(3):e0151807.

13. Sezqin AU, Punamaki RL. Perceived Changes in Social Relations after Earthquake Trauma among Eastern Anatolian Women: Associated Factors and Mental Health Consequences. Stress and Health: Journal of the International Society for the Investigation of Stress. 2016 Oct;32(4):355–366.

14. Tracy M, Norris FH, Gales S. Differences in the determinants of posttraumatic stress disorder and depression after a mass traumatic event. Depression and Anxiety. 2011;28(8):666–675.

15. Perlman SE, Friedman S, Galea S, et al. Short-term and medium-term health effects of 9/11. Lancet. 2011;378(9794):925–934.

16. Alpak G, Unal A, Bulbul F, et al. Post-traumatic stress disorder among Syrian refugees in Turkey: a cross-sectional study. International Journal of Psychiatry in Clinical Practice. 2015;19(1):45–50.

17. Mollica RF, Chernoff MC, Berthold SM, Lavelle J, Lyoo IK, Renshaw P. The mental health sequelae of traumatic head injury in South Vietnamese ex-political detainees who survived torture. Comprehensive Psychiatry. 2014;55:1626–1638.

18. Wickrama T, Wickrana KA, Banford A, Lambert J. PTSD symptoms among tsunami exposed mothers in Sri Lanka: the role of disaster exposure, culturally specific coping strategies, and recovery efforts, Anxiety, Stress and Coping. 2016 Dec 29:1–13.

19. Jefee-Bahloul H, Moustafa M, Shebl F, Barkil-Oteo A. The Yale-Kilis pilot assessment and survey of Syrian Refugees' psychological stress and openness to referral for telepsychiatry (PASSPORT Study). Telemedicine Journal and e-Health. 2014;20(10):977–979.

20. Contis G, Foley T. Depression, suicide ideation, and thyroid tumors among Ukranian adolescents exposed as children to Chernobyl radiation. Journal of Clinical Medicine Research, 2015;7(5):332–338.

21. Boscarino JA. Community disasters, psychological trauma, and crisis intervention. International Journal of Emergency Mental Health. 2015;17(1):369–371.

22. Olsen IT. Sustainability of health care: a framework for analysis. Health Policy and Planning. 1998;13(3):287–295.

23. Olteanu A, Arnberger R, Grant R, Davis C, Abramson D, Asola J. Persistence of mental health needs among children affected by Hurricane Katrina in New Orleans. Prehospital and Disaster Medicine. 2011;26(1):3–6.
24. Garshnek V, Burkle F. Applications of telemedicine and telecommunications to disaster medicine: historical and future perspectives. JAMIA. 1999;6:26–37.
25. Nicogossian AE, Doarn CR. Spacebridge to Armenia: A look back at its impact on telemedicine in disaster response. Telemedicine Journal and E Health. 2011;17(7):546–552.
26 Simmons S, Alverson D, Poropatich R, Di'Orio J, Doarn C. Applying tele-health in natural and anthropogenic disasters. Telemedicine and eHealth. 2008;14(9):968–971.
27. Yellowlees P, Burke MM, Marks SL, Hilty DM, Shore JH. Emergency telepsychiatry. Journal of Telemedicine and Telecare. 2008;14(6):277–281.
28. Reifels L, Bassilios B, Pirkis J. National telemental health responses to a major bushfire disaster. Journal of Telemedicine and Telecare. 2012;18(4):226–230.
29. US Geological Survey. Earthquake Information for 2010.
30. The World Bank. Country data, Haiti, 2015.
31. World Health Organization. Hatian Health Care: a follow up, March 2011. http://www.who.int/features/2011/haiti/en/.
32. World Health Organization. Mental Health Atlas 2011—Haiti. WHO Geneva, Switzerland. 2011.
33. Bailey RK, Bailey T, Akpudo H. On the ground in Haiti: a psychiatrist's evaluation of post-earthquake Haiti. Journal of Health Care for the Poor and Underserved. 2010;21(2):417–421.
34. McShane KM. Mental health in Haiti: a resident's perspective. Academic Psychiatry. 2011;35:1.
35. Cenat JM, Derivois D. Assessment of prevalence and determinants of posttraumatic stress disorder and depression symptoms in adult survivors of earthquake in Haiti after 30 months. Journal of Affective Disorders. 2014;159:111–117.
36. Blanc J, Bui E, Mouchenik Y, Derivois D, Birmes P. Prevalence of post-traumatic stress disorder and depression in two groups of children one year after the January 2010 earthquake in Haiti. Journal of Affective Disorders. 2015;172:121–126.
37. Louden K. Telemedicine Connects Earthquake-Ravaged Haiti to the World. Medscape Medical News. February 18, 2010.
38. Walters TJ. Deployment telemedicine: the Walter Reed Army Medical Center experience. Military Medicine. 1996;161(9):531–536.
39. Tenq JE, Thomson DR, Lascher JS, Raymond M, Ivers LC. Using mobile health (mHealth) and geospatial mapping technology in a mass campaign for reactive oral cholera vaccination in rural Haiti. Plos Neglected Tropical Diseases. 2014;8(7):e3050.
40. Freudenheim M. In Haiti, Practicing Medicine From Afar. New York Times, February 8, 2010.
41. Latifi R, Tilley EH. Telemedicine for disaster management: can it transform chaos into an organized, structured care from the distance? American Journal of Disaster Medicine. 2014;9(1):25–37.

15

Connecting the World

A Way Forward in Global Telemental Health

JUAN RODRIGUEZ GUZMAN AND ANDRES BARKIL-OTEO

Telemental health is positioning itself as an exciting and viable modality to provide access to psychiatric care in various underserved settings. This book has described several modalities of service and reviewed different telemental health models in various countries throughout the world.

We started our walk through the world of telemental health by exploring the gap between supply and demand of mental health services worldwide. We argued that telemental health is a viable option to close this gap and invited you, the reader, to think about the advantages (cost-effectiveness, efficacy, etc.) and barriers (user acceptance, resistance, legal issues, reimbursement, etc.) that come with adopting telemental health to provide care to an underserved population. We then explored how the gap in psychiatric services has led to the evolution of telemental health in various modalities: videoconferencing, store-and-forward, Web-based, and mobile telemental health. In order to understand the benefits of each of these modalities, we studied the evidence, the required technological setup, and the resources necessary for each telemental health intervention to work efficiently. Synchronous modalities (e.g., videoconferencing) are still the core of telemental health and the most studied modalities; however, the fast development of mobile technology and Internet coverage has made asynchronous modalities (store-and-forward, Web-based, and mobile telemental health) alternative methods to reach different population demographics.

We then reviewed different applications of telemental health globally. The purpose of this review was to contrast the similarities and differences between each application and to observe how unique combinations of illness burden, lack of resources, and mental health service shaped each of these models. We started with Africa, a continent where the majority of individuals with severe mental illness receive no treatment. This gap in care has been alleviated in part by telemental health partnerships between "North–South" countries (i.e., between well-resourced countries and poorly resourced countries), but "South–South" partnerships have recently increased with the rapidly falling costs of mobile telephony. South Africa is an example of what happens when a country's healthcare reforms lead to the development of national guidelines for the practice of telemental health. Not only is videoconferencing used in South Africa to provide clinical care but also it is used to provide continued medical education to clinical staff in different hospitals around the country.

The Middle East and North Africa present us with scenarios in which telemental health is seen as an option to bridge the mental health service gaps created by ongoing conflicts and political instability. According to the author, approaches to building these systems should be based on preliminary assessment of the specific cultural, financial, legal, and infrastructural needs of each country. The author notes that the countries with better ability to adopt telemental health are those with smaller mental health gaps. In countries with greater gaps, such as Syria, Iraq, and Iran, it is the author's opinion that shifting efforts from videoconferencing to less-bandwidth-demanding modules (store-and-forward or Web-based interventions) might be a feasible first step.

India presents us a with an effective and replicable mobile telemental health model for schizophrenia. In this intervention, mobile telepsychiatry clinics in conjunction with laypersons trained in mental health in villages deliver mental healthcare services in resource-poor settings. The case of Sri Lanka reminds us that for telemental health to be effective, it is necessary to have a minimum number of trained mental health staff. Telemental health redistributes existent resources, but it cannot create them without trained staff. Taiwan uses telemental health to address the long-term needs of the growing elderly population. The case of Latin America and the Caribbean provides us with an example where telehealth has taken a hold but is not currently employed as a means of increasing access to mental health services.

Telemental health has traditionally been used in middle- to high-income countries to provide care to underserved populations. Indigenous communities in Australia in most cases are geographically separated and scattered across a large landmass, thus the use of telemental health and telemedicine is seen as a possible viable alternative of providing healthcare services to communities. Denmark uses telemental health to provide care to multinational refugees via "ethnic matching." This model is designed to address language barriers and cultural disparities present in mental healthcare provision. In the United States, there is evidence to suggest that telemental health is a viable treatment model for delivering quality mental healthcare to Native American communities, where the burden of mental health conditions and difficulty accessing care continue to exist. The use of telemental health to provide care for an ethnic minority is also explored, as unique challenges arise when using telemental health across cultures. Finally, other examples of the use of telemental health include providing care in response to a disaster (e.g., Haiti earthquake) and providing care and educating clinical staff across national borders.

The future of telemental health remains exciting due to increased interest from patients and providers and rapid adoption of technology by consumers. For people with common mental disorders who want access to psychotherapeutic interventions, this technology is slowly replacing therapists with automated- or algorithm-based interventions. There are four promising modalities: computerized cognitive-behavioral therapy (cCBT), Internet-based CBT (iCBT), virtual reality exposure therapy (VRET), and mobile therapy (mTherapy). These modalities incorporate minimal clinician involvement and, in theory, could provide access to care in areas that are underserved by mental health providers. Abojoude found that published studies support the accessibility, efficiency, and reduced stigma to seek care with these technologies.[1] Both cCBT and iCBT had the most efficacy evidence while VRET and mTherapy remained promising but lacked enough research to be recommended. In the realm of mTherapy, Huguet performed a systematic review of CBT and behavioral action apps designed for depression and found that the utility of these apps is questionable.[2] Mobile apps, while highly downloaded, had low levels of adherence and no studies supporting their effectiveness. In fact, one of the main limitations telemental health will experience in the next few years is the lack of sound research to convince the scientific community, insurance companies, and policymakers of the effectiveness of these modalities. Roabinowitz highlights that most studies out there have sample sizes that are too small to make valid conclusions.[3] This author suggests that telemental health programs across the country should "join forces" in order to have sample sizes that are "sufficiently powered to detect statistical significances."[3]

In general, for the telemental health field to advance, a long term research strategy should aim to show that telemental health projects are cost effective, sustainable, and demonstrate clear improment in health outcomes. Authors have highlighted different issues with the current research conducted on telemental health. Kramer states that the lack of a standard evaluation for telemental health models is a barrier in establishing the field.[4] He suggests that a standard evaluation will not only allow researchers to "determine the impact beyond clinical outcomes" (patient satisfaction, cost effectiveness, etc.) but also stimulate research and integration of sites to power studies.[4] Cormer points out that future research should not only evaluate the overall effectiveness of telemental health but also seek to answer "when, under what circumstances, and for whom" the different modalities are most indicated.[5]

In a book on telehealth in the developing world published in 2009,[6] the authors concluded that " telemedicine does not represent 'the answer' to all public health challenges in developing countries. However, it can provide value, particularly when it is employed to strengthen and support a local team, rather than simply being used to import expertise from outside to supplement or supplant local efforts." It is clear that in the last decade since the publication of this book, telemental health success largely relied on providing valuable and needed care using local teams and expertise. Projects described in the current book could be used as models for other countries to adapt and implement to provide mental health services and to help those suffering from mental illness to take advantage of technology to seek proper care.

REFERENCES

1. Aboujaoude E, Salame W, Naim L. Telemental health: a status update. World Psychiatry. 2015;14(2):223–230.
2. Huguet A, Rao S, McGrath PJ, et al. A systematic review of cognitive behavioral therapy and behavioral activation apps for depression. PLoS One. 2016;11(5).
3. Rabinowitz T, Brennan DM, Chumbler NR, Kobb R, Yellowlees P. New directions for telemental health research. Telemedicine e-Health. 2008;14(9):972–976.
4. Kramer GM, Shore JH, Mishkind MC, Friedl KE, Poropatich RK, Gahm GA. A standard telemental health evaluation model: the time is now. Telemedicine e-Health. 2012;18(4):309–13.
5. Comer JS, Myers K. Future directions in the use of telemental health to improve the accessibility and quality of children's mental health services. Journal of Child and Adolescent Psychopharmacology. 2016;26(3):296–300.
6. Wootton R. Telehealth In The Developing World. Ottawa, ON: International Development Research Centre; 2009:299.

African TMH, 35–39
  Africa's TMH needs, 37–38
  current, 39–47
  future of, 46–47
  how other TMH experience can be
    useful for Africa, 38–39
  North-South partnerships, 34, 218
  North-South projects, 39–41, 46
  South-South partnerships, 34, 218
  South-South projects, 41–42
Alajlani, M., 81
American Indian or Alaska Native (AI/
    AN), 161. *See also* Native Americans
American Telemedicine Association
    (ATA), 25, 28, 29
apps, mobile, 25–26
"ask-the-doctor" service, 77
asylees. *See* Denmark
asynchronous (nonlive)
    communication, 31, 77
asynchronous modalities of TMH, 24, 35,
    77, 218
asynchronous TMH, 21–24
Audio Visual Assisted Therapy Aid for
    Refractory auditory hallucinations
    (AVATAR therapy), 36
Australians. *See* indigenous Australians
Aviv, A., 72t

brain injury. *See* traumatic head injury

Cameroon, 39–40
Caribbean
  history of mental illness in, 182–83
  mental health in, 182–83
  telehealth in, 184–85
  TMH in
    benefits of, 185–87
    future directions, 189–91
    limitations of, 188–89
category fallacy, 196
CCC Foundation, 111, 112t
Centers for American Indian and Alaska
    Native Health (CAIANH), 167
Cheng, T., 197
Chipps, J., 200
Clinicians' Attitudes Toward
    Telepsychiatry Questionnaire, 148, 149b
CODEC (coder/decoder system), 18
cognitive-behavioral therapy (CBT), 24,
    25, 70, 152–53, 220
community level workers (CLWs), 92, 93b,
    97, 99, 100, 102, 103
  responsibilities, 93b
  structure, 94b
  training, 93b
comorbidity, physical, 100

computerized cognitive-behavioral
    therapy (cCBT), 152–53, 220
Congo. *See* Democratic Republic of
    the Congo
connection speed, 17–18, 26–27
continuing medical education. *See*
    tele-education
Courage-Compassion-Commitment
    (CCC) project, 111, 112t
Cox, J., 197
credentialing, 171–72
cross-cultural assessments, strategies for
    overcoming linguistic discordance and
    conducting reliable, 146–47
cross-cultural TMH, 42–43, 148, 172, 193,
    200–201. *See also specific topics*
cross-cultural understanding of mental
    health, importance of, 194–96
cultural aspects in TMH,
    important, 197–98
cultural barriers. *See also* stigma associated
    with mental illness
    in development of TMH, approaching,
        199–200
    to implementation of TMH, 79–81, 172.
        See also cross-cultural TMH
        approaching, 199–200
Cultural Consultation Service in
    Canada, 195
culture-bound syndromes, 196

Deldar, K., 73t
Democratic Republic of the Congo, 40
Denmark, telepsychiatry for refugees and
    asylees in, 147–49, 151, 154–57
    international telepsychiatry, 151–53
depression, 68, 122, 204, 207, 211
    diagnostic differences and cultural
        variations, 196–97
    effects of videoconference intervention
        on depressive status, 124–25, 125t
disability benefits, 100

disasters, 203–4, 213–14. *See also* Haiti
    impact of, 204–5
    mental health consequences, 205–8
disease, defined, 194

earthquakes, 119, 204, 206, 207, 209–13
education, TMH, 40–47. *See also* psycho-
    education; tele-education
    of general public, 109–13
elderly, videoconferencing TMH program
    for the, 121–23
    qualitative outcome, 123–24
    quantitative outcome, 124–26
elderly populations, 122
    recommendations for application of
        videoconferencing in, 126–27
e-mail, 19–22, 35–36
ethical aspects of TMH, 45
ethical barriers to implementation of
    TMH, 83–84
ethnic matching, 146–47, 219
evidence-based healthcare, gap between
    knowledge and delivery of, 4–5

financial barriers to implementation of
    TMH, 84–85

Ghana, 40–41
global examples of TMH modalities for
    different utilities, 10–11t
global mental health, 4
global TMH, a way forward in, 217–21
Great East Japan Earthquake (GEJE),
    206, 207

Haiti, 210
Haiti earthquake of 2010, 204, 210
    medical and mental health
        impact, 210–12
    role of telemedicine and TMH in post-
        disaster Haiti, 212–13
head injury, traumatic, 207

health insurance, 53, 128. *See also* National
    Health Insurance
Health Professions Council of South
    Africa (HPCSA), 63, 64
HIV/AIDS, 52, 57, 59, 60
hospitalization, 20, 120, 151
hospitals, 106, 118–20, 174, 184. *See also*
    South Africa

illness, defined, 194
India, 1–2, 89
    TMH in, 89–91
        background, 91–92
        SCARF Telepsychiatry in Pudukottai
            (STEP) program, 92, 94–103
Indian Health Service, 162, 167–69, 171,
    174, 175
    Telebehavioral Health Center of
        Excellence (TBHCE), 168–70, 173
Indian Information Technology
    (Amendment) Act of 2008, 90
Indian Self-Determination and Education
    Assistance Act of 1975 (Public Law
    93-638), 168
indigenous Australians
    mental health of, 131–33
    TMH for, 134–37, 141
        barriers and potentials, 138–41
        benefits to the indigenous, 137–38
indigenous healers. *See* traditional healers
Indigenous Mental Health Team, 134
information and communications technol-
    ogy (ICT), 69, 108–9, 193
infrastructural barriers to implementation
    of TMH, 27–28, 62, 81
Integrated Services Digital Network
    (ISDN) technology, 17, 57, 62, 90, 91
"interapy," 70, 75, 76
International Society for Mental Health
    Online (ISMHO), 26, 29–30
International Telecommunications
    Union, 26

Internet. *See also specific topics*
    used for research and educational
        activities, 36–37
Internet-based cognitive-behavioral ther-
    apy (iCBT), 24, 70, 220
Internet-based interventions, 24–25
Internet connection speed, 17–18, 26–27
Internet protocol (IP) networks, 17, 41, 57,
    62, 95–96
interpreters, 146

Jiji earthquake of 1999. *See* 921
    earthquake

Kenya, 41
Kingdom of Saudi Arabia (KSA), 69
Kleinman, Arthur, 196

language barriers, 145–46
    strategies for overcoming linguistic
        discordance, 146–47
Latin America
    mental health in, 184
    telehealth in, 184–85
    TMH in
        benefits of, 185–87
        future directions for, 189–91
        limitations of, 188–89
legal aspects of TMH, 45–46
legal barriers to implementation of
    TMH, 83–84
licensure, 171
Little Prince Treatment Centre in
    Copenhagen, 148–49, 152, 154, 156
live interaction. *See* synchronous (real-
    time, live interaction) technology
local area network (LAN), 17
loneliness, effects of videoconference
    intervention on, 124–25, 125t

malpractice, 172
Marttos, Antonio C., Jr., 212

MasterMind (MAnagement of MH diSorders Through advancEd technology and seRvices—telehealth for the MIND) project, 152–53
Mazhari, S., 73t
McShane, K. M., 211
Medicaid, 174
mental health (MH), 33. *See also specific topics*
global, 4
lack of information available to people regarding, 107
"Mental Health Matters" (TV program), 43
mental health risk factors, 133
mental health services characteristics of countries from different world regions, 6–8t
mental illness, 106, 182–83. *See also specific topics*
Middle East (ME), 67–69
telemedicine in, 69–70
guideline framework for implementation of telemedicine projects, 81, 82–83b
TMH in, 70, 75–80
barriers to implementation of, 78–81, 83–85
studies of, 70, 71–74t
mobile health (mHealth), 5, 9, 27, 59–60, 96, 113, 212–13. *See also specific topics*
mobile technology, 23–24
mobile therapy (mTherapy), 77
Modai, I., 72t

National Health Insurance (NHI)
in South Africa, 51, 55, 62
in Taiwan, 117–18, 120, 121
Native American communities, 161, 176
acceptability of TMH in, 163–65
effectiveness of TMH in, 165–66
evidence supporting TMH services in, 163–66

Native American populations, implementation of TMH in, 176
barriers to, 170–72
facilitators of, 172–73
improvements and future directions, 173–76
Native Americans, 161, 176
burden of mental health issues in, 161–62
gap in access to mental health services in, 162–63
Native American telehealth programs, description of current, 167–70
921 earthquake, 119
9/11 terrorist attacks, 206–7

Olsen, I. T., 208
Ozkan, B., 73t

Pan-African eNetwork, 36, 41–43
patient satisfaction, indicators of, 152
pharmaceutical services, 120
physicians, primary care. *See* primary care physicians
post-traumatic stress disorder (PTSD), 68, 70, 167, 205–7, 211–12
primary care physicians (PCPs), 211, 213
primary healthcare (PHC) providers, 35, 38–40, 44
primary health clinics (PHCs), 53, 54, 56, 57
privacy concerns, 28–30
Psychiatric Society for Informatics (PSI), 26, 29–30
psychoeducation, 46, 76–77
psychopathological concepts, 194
psychosocial rehabilitation (PSR) services, 100, 102

Quackenbush, D. M., 74t

Rabinowitz, T., 220
real-time interaction. *See* synchronous (real-time, live interaction) technology

refugees, 204, 207. *See also* Denmark;
  Syrian refugees
regulatory issues, 30, 171–72
resource-limited settings
  challenges to implementation of TMH
    modalities in, 25
    available guidelines, 25–26
    infrastructure concerns, 27–28
    logistical concerns, 30–31
    privacy concerns, 28–30
    regulatory and legislative
      concerns, 30
    technical concerns, 26–27
  definition and scope of the term, 9
Rural and Remote Mental Health Service
  (RRMHS), 133–34
RUTE (Telemedicine University Network)
  program, 185

Sahana project, 111
San Carlos Apache Wellness Center, 174
Saudi Arabia, 69
SCARF Telepsychiatry in Pudukottai
  (STEP) program, 92, 94, 103. *See also*
  Schizophrenia Research Foundation
  achievements, 101–2
  awareness programs, 97
  challenges faced, 102–3
  consultation and treatment, 97–98
  cost of service provision, 100–101
  design and structure of the program,
    94–95, 96f
  diagnoses of the registered cases
    under, 98f
  fixed-line telepsychiatry, 95–96
  follow-up and reminders, 99–100
  medical records, 99
  mobile telepsychiatry, 96
  pharmacy, 98
  psychosocial rehabilitation, 100
schizophrenia, 76, 97, 98f
Schizophrenia Research Foundation
  (SCARF), 2. *See also* SCARF

Telepsychiatry in Pudukottai (STEP)
  program
"second-life," 77
September 11 attacks, 206–7
short message sensitive (SMS), 24,
  60, 112
sickness, defined, 194
South Africa, 51
  burden of disease, 52
  demographics, 51–52
  health system, 53–54
  mental health policy and
    legislation, 54–55
    Mental Health Care Act (2002), 54
  mobile health (mHealth) for mental
    health in, 59–60
  obstacles to telemedicine and TMH in,
    51, 61, 64, 85
    human resources, 61–62
    infrastructure, 62
    legal and ethical issues, 63–64
    political will, 62
  telemedicine for mental health in,
    57–59, 85
  telemedicine in, 51, 55–56
South Australia Rural and Remote
  Mental Health Service
  (RRMHS), 133–34
Sri Lanka
  health services in, 105
  mental health services in, 106
    barriers to accessing, 107–13
  TMH in, 109
    education of general public, 109–13
    priorities in, 109
stigma associated with mental illness, 76,
  100–103, 107, 145, 146, 185, 186, 190
  in Africa, 36, 44, 46
  reduction of, 36, 44, 46, 54, 186, 220
store-and-forward (S&F) asynchronous
  telemedicine, 9, 35
store-and-forward (S&F) technology, 5, 8,
  11t, 21–22, 75, 77

suicidal patients, telepsychiatric assessments of hospitalized, 151
suicide prevention, 112–13, 168
suicide rates, 6–8t, 106, 131–32, 162
among indigenous people, 132
supervision, 120
sustainable care
defined, 208
need for, 208
role of TMH in, 209–10
synchronous modalities of TMH, 24, 35, 218
synchronous (real-time, live interaction) technology, 9, 10t, 22–24, 148
Syria, 3–4
Syrian refugees, 74t, 75, 77–80
Syrian Telemental Health Network (STMH), 5, 8, 77

Taiwan, 117
National Health Insurance (NHI), 117–18, 120, 121
telemedicine network in, 117–18
stages in implementation of, 118–19
TMH in, 118–21
challenges facing the future for, 127–28
videoconferencing TMH program for elderly, 121–26
technical concerns and barriers to implementation of TMH, 26–27, 42–43, 81
technologies, TMH, 21–25. See also specific technologies
technology in mental healthcare provision, use of, 5
discomfort with modern technology as barrier to, 42–43
patients' perspective on, 154–56
professionals' perspective on, 153–54
Telebehavioral Health Center of Excellence (TBHCE), 168–70, 173
telecare service model, 119–21
teleclinics, 91–92, 95
telecommunication, 120
teleconsultation, 119

tele-education, 41–46, 56–59, 61, 64
Telemedicine University Network (RUTE) program, 185
telemental health (TMH). See also specific topics
barriers to implementation of, 138–41, 170–72. See also cultural barriers; stigma associated with mental illness
discomfort with modern technology, 42–43
financial, 84–85
infrastructural, 27–28, 62, 81
legal and ethical, 45–46, 83–84
technical, 26–27, 42–43, 81
cost-effectiveness, 8–9, 22–23
defined, 5
evidence for
evaluation, 19–20
specific consideration of psychiatric illness, 21
overview, 5
terminology, 5, 91
telemental health (TMH) modalities, 9
global examples of, for different utilities, 10–11t
telemental health (TMH) services, classification of, 112t
telemonitoring, 120
telepsychiatry, 91. See also specific topics
first use of the term, 34
telesupervision, 120
TMH. See telemental health
traditional healers, 38, 53–54, 107, 163
trauma. See disasters; post-traumatic stress disorder
traumatic head injury (THI), 207
tribal/telehealth outreach workers (TOWs), 164–65, 173
tuberculosis (TB), 52
Turkey, 3

Uganda, 40
United States Department of Veterans Affairs (VA), 167–68

University of Colorado Centers for
    American Indian and Alaska Native
    Health (CAIANH), 167

Veterans Affairs (VA). *See* United States
    Department of Veterans Affairs
videoconferencing (VC), 34, 148
videoconferencing-based TMH
    (VC-TMH), 15–16. *See also* elderly,
    videoconferencing TMH program
    for the
    access to patient medical record, 19
    audio quality, 17

basic set-up, 16
network connection, 17
video quality, 17–19
"virtual mental health clinic," 20
virtual reality exposure therapy (VRET),
    77, 220
"virtual reality psychotherapy," 76–78

Wagner, B., 71t, 72t